From leaders in every area of health care,
praise for

THE AMERICAN WAY OF HEALTH

"A very complicated and timely subject presented in a clear and balanced way. Highly readable, a superb contribution."

> —David B. Skinner, M.D., President
> The New York Hospital–Cornell Medical Center

"The first consumer-friendly, understandable analysis of the current national health-reform quagmire, highly recommended to all who are concerned about the nation's health and / or their own."

> —John C. Lewin, M.D., Director
> Department of Health, State of Hawaii

"A down-to-earth description of our up-in-the-air health-care system."

> —Thomas O. Pyle, CEO
> MetLife HealthCare

"Defines the central issues for the lay reader in understandable terms. Gives normal Americans the information they need to make their own diagnosis and prescribe their own treatment, based on their own needs. It will expand the debate to those who must live with the consequences."

—Brent C. James, M.D., M.Stat., Executive Director
IHC Institute for Health Care Delivery Research

"Valuable and timely, it brings together a clear view of the human concerns in health care and a wealth of information about the state of American health-care delivery."

—David M. Lawrence, M.D., Chairman and CEO
Kaiser Permanente

"The most comprehensive examination of a complex subject presented in terms everyone can understand."

—Alan R. Nelson, M.D., Executive Vice-President
American Society of Internal Medicine, former
President, American Medical Association

THE AMERICAN WAY
OF HEALTH

THE AMERICAN WAY OF HEALTH

*How Medicine Is Changing and
What It Means to You*

JANICE CASTRO

BACK
BAY
BOOKS

Little, Brown and Company

Boston   New York   Toronto   London

First Edition

Library of Congress Cataloging-in-Publication Data

Castro, Janice.
    The American way of health: How Medicine Is Changing and What It Means to You / Janice Castro. — 1st ed.
        p.   cm.
    Includes index.
    ISBN 0-316-13272-1 (hc)
    ISBN 0-316-13275-6 (pb)
    1. Health care reform — United States.   2. Medical care, Cost of — United States.   3. Medical economics — United States.   I. Title.
RA395.A3C39   1994
362.1'0973 — dc20   94-5949

HC: 10 9 8 7 6 5 4 3 2 1
PB: 10 9 8 7 6 5 4 3 2 1

MV-NY

Published simultaneously in Canada
by Little, Brown & Company (Canada) Limited

Printed in the United States of America

For Hugh Pickett and Ronald P. Kriss

CONTENTS

THANKS

FIRST of all, to my father, for his example of courage during several close calls. And for all those conversations at dawn.

I literally could not have written this book without the enthusiastic support of *Time* managing editor Jim Gaines, who readily freed me from my health-care reporting responsibilities during President Clinton's busy first year so that I could focus on this project. I am indebted to John Stacks, deputy managing editor of *Time*, who got me started and even offered me his home in Ireland as a writer's haven; to Bernie Baumohl, *Time* assistant editor, and my friend Sanford Teller, whose spontaneous help in the research contributed enormously; and to my colleagues Michael Duffy and Dick Thompson for their collaboration in decoding The Plan.

Whatever reporters understand, they learn from people who know more than they ever will about subjects like this. I am deeply grateful to Dr. Paul Ellwood for his generous and unstinting help; to Dr. Robert Brook and Dr. Brent James for their insights on medical quality and physician motivation; to Dr. David Skinner, chief executive of New York Hospital, Dr. Jack Lewin, director of Hawaii's medical system, and Dr. Robert Waller and his astute colleagues at the Mayo Clinic for their plainspoken candor on the promise and the limits of medicine; to Wayne Isom, a top heart surgeon who let me follow him in and out of operating rooms; to Dr. James Todd, John Crosby, Kirk Johnson, Dr. Roy Schwarz, and the other helpful people at the American Medical Association; and to Professors Alain Enthoven of Stanford, William Baumol of New York University, and Uwe Reinhardt of Princeton for their guidance on the economics.

I'm also grateful to many people who shared their personal medical experiences with me so that I could learn, especially John Comer, Howard Godnick, and Father Edward Larkin, as well as countless nurses, physicians, health providers, and public officials who helped me understand their parts of health care, in particular Rick Scott, Dr. Malcolm Rothbard, Dr. Albert Bernstein, Tom Pyle, Diane Jones, Dr. William Rodney, Judith Miller Jones, and Ronda Kotelchuck; to Michael Ovitz, for his encouragement; to my brother, Jim, Howard and Pat Gates, and Mona Janopaul for theirs; to John Gallagher, Adam and Allegra Honigman, and Ken Baierlein, who helped more than they knew; and to Jim Silberman, an editor any writer would be lucky to have. And finally, to Ebony Britton, Matthew Rodriguez, and Aaron Moore, for whom, in a very real sense, this book was written.

THE AMERICAN WAY
OF HEALTH

1

BASIC PRINCIPLES

ASK most people what they think about the state of American medicine, and they will tell you about their own doctors, or about something that happened to them during an illness. Chances are, if they see a need for health-care change, it will be very specific, based on personal experience.

On the other hand, listen to American leaders discussing health-care reform. They speak of providers. Access. Alliances. Competition. Mandates. What in Heaven's name are they talking about? The concepts seem impossibly complicated and remote from the experience of one sick person needing help. But while discussions of health-care reform may be bewildering, listen closely: they are talking about you and your needs.

This book will help the general reader understand how the American health system works, why it costs so much, and why we are suddenly embroiled in an argument over how to make profound changes in everyone's private medical arrangements.

Medicine is too important, too personal, to be left to economists and politicians. Any broad national reform is going to affect every American. After all, the health-care debate is really about life and death. It is about those times when people need help and about whether it will be there, about one sick patient at a time and the doctor or nurse who provides care. Buried in all of the technical talk are two simple questions: how should that person be helped, and who will pay the bill?

Health-care reform is much more than an arcane economic policy debate, more than a political issue.

It is fundamentally a moral problem.

Viewed in that light, the challenge of health-care reform begins to come more clearly into focus. It is not really that complicated.

We know what we need to do.

We need to take care of old people when they can no longer take care of themselves. Children should see doctors and dentists. A pregnant woman should be able to check in with a doctor as the baby grows. People should not be dying in the street. Mentally ill Americans should not be wandering around, scavenging in garbage cans and sleeping in cardboard boxes. They are not someone else's problem. They are us. Families shouldn't lose their homes over the cost of coping with medical disasters. Breadwinners should not quit good jobs in order to qualify for poor people's insurance. Those with high incomes should contribute more to the cost of their care. People should take responsibility for their own health and for their family's. Children should not be having children. Companies should not force people out because they might get expensive illnesses. Insurance companies should not dump you when you get sick. Medical care should make you feel better.

Most of these principles can be addressed to some extent in a sound and equitable medical system that ensures access to basic care for all Americans. But meeting many of these needs also requires moral responsibility, by patients and doctors, employers and parents, and everyone else in the American family. No government program can make us better people. No financing system can guarantee quality or enforce personal responsibility for oneself, one's own family, and fellow citizens. "I don't see health care as a right," says Stuart Orsher, a Manhattan internist, "not, I mean, as something that should be available on demand. I see it as something like national defense or fire and police protection. In a civilized society, you should not expect to be shot on the street; the fire department should come when your house is burning; and doctors should not turn their backs on you when you are in need."

If we are going to ensure that every American has access to decent health care, while also controlling the burgeoning costs, all of us must curb our medical greed. All of us must stop pretending that someone else is paying the bills. "What do you think most people would say if one of their parents called up and said they needed a hundred and twenty-five thousand dollars for an operation?" asks one economist. "Do you think that son or daughter would think twice and wonder whether that operation was really necessary? Of course they would. But none of us think we pay for medical care. And of course we all do."

All of us must pay our share. We must also stop the violence and self-destruction. When adolescents shoot children in the back, doctors can only do so much. When a friend gets drunk and plows into a family driving home, the emergency room cannot make them whole.

Something is wrong, and medicine cannot fix it. There is no magic economic formula. There are no guarantees. Our political leaders may argue for the next year or two about how best to rearrange American health care. But no set of rules and no system of financing can legislate compassion or moral rectitude.

*   *   *

In a remote rural hospital in Texas, a young veterinarian is sitting at a table, trying to decide what to do. She was helping a cow through a difficult delivery when the cow slammed her into a fence, severing most of her right middle finger. The finger has been put on ice.

Here's her problem: because she recently left her old job in the city and moved here to set up her practice, her new insurance policy has not yet taken effect. This is a poor town, where the doctor and the veterinarian are sometimes paid with a gracious invitation to dinner. The doctor says that a few months back, a poor patient showed his gratitude by sharing a slug from a prized bottle locked away for special occasions. The vet doesn't have much in the way of savings or prospective revenue. The operation to reattach her finger will cost more than $400. For less than $100, of course, they can just sew up the stump. She's the only vet in a town full of horses, cattle, and other animals. She is needed here. Doing without that finger will affect her ability to make a living, will make it harder, for example, to perform veterinary surgery. But $400 is an awful lot of money.

She's thinking it might be better to do without the finger. Her doctor is not offering to do without the fee.

A nurse in Manhattan has had it up to here with what she sees every day. Sloppy doctors who seem immune to reproach, and other doctors and nurses, decent and hard-pressed, who can barely keep pace with the avalanche of problems tumbling through the doors of her hospital. Drug addicts who have learned how to game the Medicaid system, collecting room and board in the hospital for several days by asserting their right to refuse a simple outpatient procedure. Sick and frightened old people who have worked hard all of their lives, who have not had a proper pair of eyeglasses in years and can barely hear, trying to ask questions about their medications of an impatient and overworked emergency room staff. Crack babies, some of whom have been abandoned, who are now being subjected to massive medical intervention by doctors and nurses battling to save them — for what kind of life? Their best hope is often severe disability and retardation and life in an institution.

Across the street from the hospital where this nurse works is a halfway house for teenage mothers. The girls sit outside talking and eating junk food. Most of them have babies and are already pregnant again. There are about a dozen trash cans on that corner, but they drop their food wrappers and soda cans on the ground. "Where is the pride?" the nurse asks. "Where are their families? What is going to happen to those children? Children shouldn't be having children. They shouldn't be allowed to have children until they are ready to love them and take care of them."

A frail old man lies on a gurney in a central California emergency room. He was recently released from the hospital after major surgery, and now he's back. He lives alone. He is barely conscious. The doctor in charge of the emergency room impatiently asks him whether he has been taking his pills. The old man whispers that, since his operation, he has been so weak that he cannot remember which pills he is supposed to take. The doctor begins shouting at him. The same doctor approaches an extremely ill, elderly woman across the room. She is slumped in a wheelchair, waiting for help. "Did you have a nice Christmas?" he asks. "Yes," she replies. "Good, because you won't live to see another one."

A physician in Los Angeles describes the patient he has just released from UCLA Medical Center after a couple of weeks of intensive treatment. "He was a Skid Row alcoholic. Of course we helped him. We did our best. But I can't get him out of my mind. In the last few weeks we spent more than a hundred thousand dollars cleaning him up, fixing him up, trying to make him better. And you know where he is right now? Back on Skid Row. We'll see him again, if he lives long enough. We can't fix his life. How come we are willing to devote all of these medical resources to saving people once they have nearly killed themselves, when we can't seem to find a way to get them off Skid Row?"

A dentist finishes up a minor repair for a longtime patient, then makes a surprising offer. The bill is $100. The patient's insurance covers 70 percent of the bill. The patient will get back $70; the visit will cost her $30.

"Make the check for a hundred and ten," says the dentist, "and I'll give you a bill for a hundred and thirty."

That way, the patient can get back $91. The visit will cost her $19. The dentist will make an extra $10.

Together, they commit a little fraud, adding 30 percent to the insurance bill.

At the Los Angeles Free Clinic, which offers free medical care to everyone regardless of income, no questions asked, a woman waits to see a doctor. Her ten-year-old son sits with her. Will he have a checkup too? "Oh no!" she says. "He has never been to the doctor! He's not old enough."

In Manhattan, a visiting nurse makes house calls all over town, taking care of the ailing elderly, people with AIDS, diabetics who have had their feet amputated, and others who are homebound. She checks their blood pressure, blood sugar levels, temperature, and other vital signs. She dresses their wounds, asks them how they are sleeping, how they feel in general. She administers medications, adjusting the dosage if necessary, and makes sure they know how to take them. She visits elderly women with osteoporosis, giving them injections to help build up their bone strength. She reports disturbing signs of trouble to her patients' physicians, sometimes increasing the frequency of her visits for a while when a patient suffers a setback. She visits newborn babies who are in danger of abuse or neglect. She even visits middle-class mothers who are simply afraid that they do not know how to care for their first child.

If her patients are covered by Medicare or Medicaid, those programs pay for her visits, up to a point. Other patients pay out of pocket for her services (as much as $110 per visit), or are covered for a few visits under their own insurance policies. For many seriously ill patients, she is the only one who comes to check on them. Often, though, she cannot visit them until an escort is available to accompany her into their neighborhoods, especially at night. If she went alone, her life would be in danger. Part of the cost of providing a visiting nurse — and part of the reason her availability to assist the helpless is therefore limited — is the necessary expense of protecting her from violence.

A physical therapist in her early thirties is expecting her first child. She is well insured. She is healthy. She has received good advice on proper nutrition. She has had all of the diagnostic tests that medicine offers. She is under the care of an obstetrician and will deliver her baby in a major teaching hospital. Now it is up to her and to fate. But she is not satisfied. "If one little finger is wrong," she says, "I'm going to sue that guy!"

A New York doctor mentions one of his patients, a famous man who is a member of one of the richest families in the country. The patient is on Medicare.

On any given day, some of the wealthiest Americans submit their medical bills to Medicare. Taxpayers, many of whom are uninsured, help to pay those bills.

*   *   *

In San Francisco, a billing manager for a leading teaching hospital remembers the patient who called to protest an enormous bill charging him for a kidney transplant. He insisted that he hadn't had one. The billing staff insisted he had. They had the paperwork right there. The patient pointed out that he was a patient in a special research program for liver transplants. He said they don't give kidneys to people in that program. They said he was mistaken and sternly warned him to pay the bill.

The manager remembers the family that called to question a bill for major surgery. The date of the surgery was more than a month after the patient had died. "It happens all the time. People get charged for things they never got." She tells of another patient who kept calling to say his insurance bills did not make any sense and asking for help in sorting them out. He was getting nowhere. Finally, they had to evacuate the offices one night in the summer of 1993 when he called and said he was going to blow up the place. She remembers the night her father died. The next day, the hospital began calling her mother and threatening to take action for late payment of the bills. Her mother pointed out the date of death and promised to pay. The hospital kept calling and threatening to sue. That's when the young woman decided to work in hospital administration. Somebody had to do a better job; this should not happen to people like her mother.

A doctor in Hawaii recalls the drug addict who hit the emergency room late one night and was refusing treatment for at least one gaping bullet wound. The physician rushed in to help. "I was insisting that he needed medical care. I reached down to look at the laceration I could see, and suddenly there was a gun at my temple. We were nose to nose. He had these big starey eyes. He said he was going to kill me. I lost it. I started screaming at him, telling him he could just fucking die where he was, because he didn't have the brains to accept help when it was being offered. He stared at me, with this gun still jammed against my temple. I didn't care. I dared him to go ahead and shoot. I was fed up. He got this weird look on his face and he put the gun down. He said, 'You're crazy!' Maybe I am. What the hell are we supposed to do?"

What indeed? Guaranteeing medical coverage to all Americans will not solve all of the problems that our medical system is asked to handle. It will not make us healthier. Americans must stop blaming medicine for everything that goes wrong with their health. And it is time for patients to understand that when medicine is unsuccessful, it does not always mean that a doctor has committed malpractice.

Having insurance will do nothing to curb drug abuse, which cost the United States an estimated $67 billion in 1990 in medical treatment and other related expenses.[1] Studies show that half of all people arrested for major crimes, including homicide, theft, and assault, were using illegal drugs at the time.[2] Insurance will not make Americans more responsible about alcohol abuse, which cost the country $99 billion in 1990.[3] It will not prevent the 11 million U.S. highway crashes every year that take some 40,000 lives; one-third of those collisions are caused by excessive speed, and many are caused by drinking.[4] It will not take the automatic weapons out of the hands of teenagers. Every day in America, 4,900 teenagers become the victims of violent assaults.[5]

Guaranteeing coverage will not make immoral people better parents. It will not encourage irresponsible parents to get their children the vaccinations that are readily available to them. Every day in the United States, 2,700 teenage girls become pregnant and 1,300 give birth. Families must take responsibility. Every day, 2,500 teenagers drop out of school, plunging into a lifetime of postindustrial pove-

Nor does having insurance mean that you can get to a doctor in time if you live in any one of hundreds of small towns or the broad swaths of rural America that stretch for hundreds of square miles where there are no doctors. America needs more doctors who want to take care of families, even those living in isolated or impoverished areas. Medicine is not always just, not always kind. It should be. Guaranteeing coverage will not make callous doctors compassionate or encourage selfish relatives to visit their ailing elders more often. Federal mandates do not change human behavior. Responsible people do.

Americans need to face the tough decisions about how to allocate medical resources more sensibly. They need to think about how to know when to let people go. They also need to face the fact that, too often, families are ready to let someone go before the patient is ready to die. It is all too easy to blame doctors and hospitals for "wasting" money on heroic intervention at the end of life. It is easy to cite figures about all of the money spent providing care during the last six months of life. But when, exactly, do the last six months of a life start?

There are no easy answers. Every discussion about such questions seems to feature a hypothetical eighty-five-year-old man who has smoked three packs of cigarettes and downed a fifth of vodka every day of his life and now wants a heart transplant. Around America's dinner tables, everyone seems ready to decide that this man must forgo the transplant so that children can have vaccinations. The equation is nonsensical. It is not that simple. The choices are seldom clear.

American medical science has now reached a level of expertise and skill where it can do much more than we can afford to guarantee to everyone in every case.

A health plan that seems to promise that we can have it all is ducking the truth. But where do we draw the line? Who decides?

We can no longer afford to think of medicine as some sort of space-age body shop. We can no longer expect the government or some other entity to pay for every physical treatment we think we need or to intervene at all costs to prevent death and decay. Nor can we continue to avoid moral responsibility for the decisions we keep shifting to medicine. We can't keep blaming the Special Interests. When it comes to health services, we are all Special Interests. It is time to have a national heart-to-heart about medical rights and responsibilities and about the social contract.

Oregon has done it, in a town-by-town, wrenching community discussion over which medical problems the state can promise to pay for, which needs are greatest, and, hardest of all, when some results are worth more than others. That hypothetical eighty-five-year-old is out of luck if he lives in Oregon. But the decisions faced by the people of that state were far more subtle and difficult than that. The people of Oregon have painstakingly decided when to say no, so that they will have the ability to care for their children and for people who have a decent chance of resuming a relatively healthy life. Even at that, the state is not sure it will be able to find the money to pay for its hard-won compromises on the promise of medicine.

No other state — no other nation — has ever undertaken such a process. European health leaders, facing difficult decisions themselves about how to ration medical care more severely than ever before, visit Oregon to learn how its people did it. They've never had to discuss rationing in public, though they have been doing it. Now that they must, they want to learn from the people who faced the hard choices.

No one comes from Washington, D.C.

Until the United States is willing to engage in such a probing national dialogue, the strain on our capacity to deal with all social problems will grow.

* * *

"In medicine, we talk about the quandary we face when a man jumps off a cliff and is floundering in the water," muses Jane Campion, an administrative nurse at the Mayo Clinic. "And a second man is standing at the edge of the cliff, trying to decide whether to jump. Whom do you save? We are always drawn to the drama of saving the man in the water. But he has already made his decision. If you can only save one of them, what about the man on the cliff, who is still trying to decide what to do?"

But how do you know when you can only save one of them? How do you know the man on the cliff will jump, and whose fault is it if he does? It is not the job of medicine to make decisions about how to treat the man in the water based on how he got there. That is the job of the society. Medicine's job is to know everything it can about what happens to an injured man struggling in deep water and what it will take to restore him to the best possible health. Society's job is to decide how to pay for it.

The essential message of health reform is that for the majority of Americans, who are well insured, the party's over. No more "free" medical coverage, with an insurance company automatically paying almost any bill a patient sends to it. Many people already know this; their health coverage has come under some restrictions if, for instance, they have joined health maintenance organizations. The restrictions are going to grow tighter.

No matter which national plan for health reform prevails — even if reform stalls and no broad new health law is passed — most Americans are going to pay more in the coming years to get less in health care. That does not necessarily mean that they will get less than they need. But the days of unlimited access to medical services are over. Some people will be better off than they are now; many will not.

The only real issue is how we are going to organize the cut-backs.

We can preserve, even enhance, the quality of medicine while curbing the price. But will we? The following chapters will help readers understand what is at stake in the health debate, and the choices they face.

2

BEGINNINGS

"COME on now, Gail, push through it! You can do it! Push! Harder!"

Gail Rodriguez, thirty-eight, has been in labor since early this morning at the Kaiser Permanente hospital in Walnut Creek, California. Several hours ago, she was given an injection to reduce the pain. It helped. But now, at 6:05 P.M., she is so exhausted that she is having trouble pushing hard enough to give birth. Heidi Olander, the ob-gyn resident on duty tonight, decided a few moments ago that Gail needs help to bring this baby into the world. She has rushed Rodriguez into Delivery Room 2 and is now unwrapping a special vacuum device that will provide extra suction during the next contraction. As the last contraction passed, everyone in the delivery room relaxed for a moment. Now they spring into action as the next one begins. Gail rises half off the table, her shoulders curling forward with the force of her effort.

"Come on, that's great! Keep pushing! Come on!"

Gail's husband, Joe, is supporting her back, helping her to hold the crunch position when each contraction comes, her knees up, her upper body lifting. His sister, Patty, is holding Gail's right hand and murmuring encouragement. A stereo speaker relays audio signals from the fetal monitor that measures the baby's rapid heartbeat, which is pounding along at roughly twice the normal adult pulse. It sounds like an Australian wobble-board: "VoooomPAHpah! Vooom-PAHpah! VooomPAHpah!" With each contraction, the baby whose heartbeat fills the room surges a tiny bit closer to birth.

"Keep pushing! Keep pushing!"

6:09 P.M.: As the next contraction comes, Olander employs the vacuum gadget, which, quite frankly, works something like a plumber's helper. She gently places its soft concave top against the top of the baby's head, which is now just visible at the opening of his mother's body. Olander tugs mightily, pulling as Rodriguez pushes. The vacuum device makes a loud sucking noise as it pulls away from the baby's moist head. Olander puts it in place again, pulling hard.

"Come on, Gail! It's really close! Go for it!"

Dr. Dennis Randall, the obstetrician on duty, has arrived. He stands behind Olander, leaning forward, his hands on his hips, in case she needs help. He's in a restless, chatty mood. "I don't know why I'm here. I'm just wondering if you need me at all, Heidi." Olander is too busy to respond. Just then, Olander's beeper goes off. Randall makes himself useful. As Olander tugs, he reaches around under her surgical gown to remove the beeper that is clipped to her belt. He moves to a wall phone away from this circle of frantic activity to retrieve her message, the most-skilled medical person in the room acting as his resident's secretary.

"Come on, push through it! Push through it! You're almost there!"

The baby's head is still visible, but it has not come any farther forward this time. The contraction passes.

Olander's voice is soothing. She pats Rodriguez on the leg. "Okay, Gail, don't worry, you're doing fine. You're doing fine. We'll wait for the next contraction."

Rodriguez releases what sounds like all of the breath in her body, gaining a brief moment of respite. She and her husband have been trying to have this baby for seven years. After two years of infertility therapy, she was able to conceive last January.

6:11: The next contraction has started. The baby's head is now beginning to emerge, inch by inch, easing forward, then sliding almost all the way back.

6:13: "OK! It's coming!" Rodriguez is pushing for all she's worth. The top of the baby's head surges forward an inch or two, then recedes an inch.

6:14: "Come on, push! Matthew is right there!" Gail cries out, putting all of her strength into it.

6:16: "Do it! Do it! You're almost there! Come on, Gail, keep it up! He's coming!"

At 6:18, as casually as if he hadn't realized they were waiting for him, Matthew Rodriguez thrusts his curly red head into the world and opens his huge blue eyes wide, turning his face from side to side and taking in this noisy crew. "Push, Gail!" In one smooth movement, Olander swiftly pulls him all the way out and lays him on his mother's chest for a moment. Joe begins to cry, resting his hand ever so gently on his son's back. Gail looks as if she can't believe it's over. Matthew is making happy gurgling noises, his eyes bright and focused. He never does cry. As his father leans close, cooing along with his mother, Matthew's eyes follow their voices, looking from one to the other, right, left, right, left. He looks unaccountably wise.

Olander scoops him up, clamps and cuts the cord, and weighs him.

"Seven pounds, eight ounces! I think he needs to go to the nursery for a little while. See how juicy he is?" Olander is using a small blue suctioning device, removing tiny amounts of fluid from Matthew's mouth and nose.

"Don't worry, this is normal. This is normal. Look how pink he is!"

A nurse wraps Matthew in swaddling clothes under a warming lamp on a small table that is behind the delivery bed. Olander hovers protectively over him, touching him, using the suction device, as Gail twists around to watch.

It isn't always this hard. Earlier, Regina Britton was in delivery barely ten minutes, encouraged by her husband, Tony, and her sister, Tina, before Ebony Michelle was born. Announcing his daughter's name, a beaming Tony added: "Her big brother Justin named her!"

Ebony has two older brothers. Antonio, Jr., was the first to come along, seven years ago, when Regina was twenty and Tony was twenty-two. Justin was born four years later. The Brittons have decided not to have any more babies. "It's so hard to raise kids right these days," said Tina. "And we are going to do it right!" added Tony. He was beside himself, gazing at his wife and daughter: "Happy birthday, little girl. I'm so happy, oh honey, I'm so happy." Then he was out the door and back before Regina even left the delivery room. "I reached everybody! All of the grandparents are getting ready to come over!"

Out at the nurses' station after Ebony was born, Dr. Joel Cohen, a Kaiser obstetrician helping out on this particularly busy weekend, was in a reflective mood. "There's a lot of heartache and pain in medicine, you know? But ob-gyn is a happy field. I love my work." He said his first ambition in life was to be an archaeologist. "Then I decided I wanted to be an astronaut. After my freshman year at the University of Pittsburgh, though, I knew I wanted to be a doctor. I wanted to help people."

*   *   *

6:34 P.M.: As Gail Rodriguez is wheeled out of Delivery Room 2 to the recovery area down the hall, Anna Moore is being whisked into Delivery Room 1. Someone at the nurses' station is making popcorn. Everyone is happy about Matthew. This is a busy labor ward, yet every baby born here puts smiles on the faces of the doctors and nurses for a few minutes. "He's so lively!" says one nurse: "Feel it? Do you feel that adrenaline?"

In each of these two delivery rooms, the only ones at Kaiser's Walnut Creek hospital, some thirty miles east of San Francisco, two thousand babies are born every year. Four thousand new Californians. Four thousand new American citizens, one out of every thousand infants being born this year in the new American Baby Boom that is underway. Many are first-generation Americans, their parents recent arrivals from Asia, Central or South America, occasionally Eastern Europe. Every time, a nurse takes out a big green ledger that would look right at home in a 1940 Clark Gable movie and records the birth with a ballpoint pen. She carefully draws a line across two wide pages, about an inch below the last line, and notes thirty-four separate pieces of information, from the birth position and any complications to the baby's weight and sex. To look up any of this information and draw any broad conclusions, a researcher would have to pull out one of these huge ledgers for each hospital, one for every year. At the front of this year's ledger, someone has written down the total births at the hospital for each year since it opened in 1953 (when 749 babies were born).

The Kaiser hospital in Walnut Creek looks nothing like the average big-city medical center. Spread out in a parklike campus, its low-slung units connected by winding paths that meander under the trees, it seems more like a suburban high school at first glance. Most of the private rooms open onto small, peaceful patios, each with its own flowers and patch of lawn. But with ten or eleven babies beginning their lives here every day, the labor wing jumps. Up and down the halls as Gail Rodriguez was giving birth, other expectant mothers waited in their tiny labor rooms. One, expecting her first baby, had been in labor for more than eight hours. All day, her young husband came and went, each time returning with a big smile, each time more marinated than when he left. The nurses began speculating about whether he would be conscious by the time his son was born. The next time he came weaving in, about dinnertime, a nurse handed him a mug of coffee and a plate of nachos, pointed at a chair, and told him to eat.

This homey little hospital is Kaiser's principal Bay Area birthing center, serving families in a hundred-mile radius, from the Sonoma wine country a couple of hours north, to Silicon Valley to the west, to the peach orchards and turkey farms of Turlock down in the Central Valley southeast of here. Starting in the 1970s, thanks largely to the explosive growth of Silicon Valley, Walnut Creek was transformed virtually overnight from a small rural town to a sprawling bedroom community. Because it was convenient to so many towns, Walnut Creek also became a medical center.

Since 1975, the rate of births at Kaiser Walnut Creek has more than doubled, from 1,800 per year to the current 4,000. Just since 1987, the rate has picked up by a third, from 3,071 that year. Sometimes it seems as though they're all being born the same night. Says one doctor: "Full moons, oh please! A couple of days ago, the night before the full moon, we had three sets of premature twins and one set of premature triplets. Something to do with the tides. It happens every time. Just before a big storm, when the barometric pressure drops, we always get more babies than usual. You explain it."

Ironically, this town where so many lives begin is also a bustling haven for those whose lives are ending. Retirement is a major industry in Walnut Creek, thanks to the transportation advantages that make it a convenient place to visit Mom and Dad. Hospitals, private housing complexes for the elderly, nursing homes, medical equipment suppliers, and other facilities serving the well-to-do aged continue to expand under the shade of oak trees and along the rolling hills here. It is not unusual, driving down these sunny streets, to see people in their eighties driving motorized carts or pushing special bicycle-style walkers equipped with outsized shopping baskets along the sidewalks. In a sense, Walnut Creek has evolved in less than thirty years from a farming community to a managed-care town, whether in the form of Kaiser's group practice services or the bustling and lucrative business of the profit-making firms that have come here to serve the Medicare population.

Kaiser helped pioneer managed care in the United States. When its prepaid health plan was introduced in the late 1930s for Kaiser's construction, steel, and shipyard workers, the Oakland, California–based company was blasted for socializing medicine. Under the Kaiser plan, doctors managed large group practices, providing whatever care a worker or family member needed for a fixed monthly fee and keeping an eye on the budget. Criticized as assembly-line care, the plan nevertheless won broad popularity with California families once it began to sign up non-Kaiser workers at the end of World War II.

Accusations linger that prepaid health plans are socialist. Physicians say that such programs destroy their independence. In a sense, they are right, but it is more accurate to describe the movement toward prepaid plans as the large-scale displacement of small-town retailers by the Wal-Marts of medicine. The Kaiser program is run by doctors following entrepreneurial instincts, offering one-stop medical shopping, convenience, and low prices to families that usually are perfectly free to opt instead for old-fashioned relationships with physicians in private practice.

The growth of such plans was probably inevitable, even though something important was lost in the process, in particular, close personal relationships with a doctor who answered all of a family's needs. Medicine was changing. Its knowledge and skills were expanding exponentially. Doctors were no longer capable of knowing everything that "medicine" knew, and so they specialized. As families consulted more and more specialists, the family doctor increasingly acted as the traffic controller, sending patients to colleagues more knowledgeable about the problem of the moment.

Participation in prepaid health plans, which usually offered the full range of medical specialties, grew along with the postwar pressures on American families. By the early 1980s, most parents were working outside the home. For many families, time had become even more precious than money. The right to drive all over town — or, more likely in California, to several towns — to visit internists, pediatricians, gynecologists, and other specialists was losing its charm. A growing number of families were willing to give up unlimited choice of their own doctors for the lower costs and convenience of Kaiser's shopping-mall approach to medicine, especially in the western states, where the distances are greater. As babies are born in Walnut Creek, for example, nurses ask the mothers which Kaiser center is most convenient to their home or office, then assign the baby a pediatrician and book appointments for visits. Do the mothers resent having a pediatrician assigned to them? "No," says one new mother in Walnut Creek. "I feel safer. The Kaiser doctors are pretty good, and they handle all of the paperwork. The only thing that bothers me is that lots of times you have to wait several weeks for an appointment.

But if you're really sick, you can see someone that day."
Someone? Anyone? "Well, yeah, whoever is available."

Medicine has become too complicated for most Americans to understand. Plans like Kaiser's relieve patients of the nagging sense of incompetence as medical consumers. The managed-care movement that started in the West is now taking over the eastern half of the United States. Many families find they don't mind giving up some personal choice in exchange for the convenience and predictable costs. In a *Time*/CNN poll conducted by Yankelovich Partners in September 1993, 57 percent of those surveyed said that a requirement to join a managed-care health plan would not be an excessive infringement on their freedom to choose a doctor.

Now the largest independent American health plan, Kaiser delivers more than $10 billion in medical services each year, accounting for about 1 percent of all U.S. medical spending. The Kaiser program serves more than 6.6 million members in sixteen states, from Hawaii to Massachusetts, as well as the District of Columbia. The plan employs nearly ten thousand doctors, 57 percent of whom are family practitioners, and offers comprehensive benefits, from routine checkups to hospitalization and surgery.

In Kaiser's Walnut Creek hospital, most of the babies are delivered by midwives. Many mothers prefer midwives. Because they seem less clinical and formal than physicians, the mothers find it easier to relax during the effort of giving birth. JoAnn Jackson is the midwife on duty tonight. "You don't need to be in a hospital to do this," Jackson scoffs. "You could do this in a tent! Most births are perfectly normal. You know why we're here? Because the California Medical Association won't allow midwives to deliver babies unless they are in a hospital. Kaiser saves money by using us, you know. This way, they don't need as many doctors and nurses." Maybe so, but the doctors and nurses are there when they are needed.

7:23 P.M.: In Delivery Room 1, Anna Moore has been on the verge of having her baby for nearly an hour. The baby's head is now visible. Anna pushes hard — one, two, three times. The baby begins to emerge, facedown, then suddenly stops. It is wedged tightly at the opening of Anna's body. "Oh my God, the shoulder's stuck!" JoAnn is tugging at the baby's head, turning it from side to side. It won't budge. "The shoulder's stuck!"

Bang! The door flies open, hitting an equipment cart, as Heidi, a pediatrician, and two nurses rush into the room to help. Together, they quickly get the baby out.

7:25: "It's a boy! Oh, God, it's a little boy!" At the warming table, the pediatrician is working rapidly on Aaron Michael Moore, suctioning liquids from his mouth. She turns to a nurse, speaking in low, commanding tones: "Call Nursery 1. Tell them a baby's coming! Grunting, respiratory distress." The doctor touches Anna's arm: "Don't worry. This is a normal procedure, perfectly normal. I just want to check his oxygen status." But this is not an ordinary birth. Cradling the baby and trailed by his worried father, the pediatrician rushes out of the delivery room and down the hall to the pediatric intensive care unit.

Fortunately for Aaron Moore, he was not born in a tent. After a short time in intensive care, he was able to go home, in perfect health. It is true that most births are normal, almost routine. But just in case, Kaiser's pediatric intensive care unit is only twenty to thirty steps from the delivery rooms.

Matthew, Ebony, and Aaron are from slightly different backgrounds. Matthew's parents are human resources managers, his dad for Circuit City and his mom for Pacific Bell.

Ebony's dad is a carpenter. Aaron's is an electrical engineer for a firm that builds submarine communications systems for the Navy; his mom works at a print shop. But these three infants have something important in common, something that none of us has ever had. Not their parents, not their grandparents or their aunts or uncles or cousins, not their pediatricians or their nurses or midwives. They were born in September 1993, the month that President Bill Clinton outlined his proposal to overhaul the American medical system. And no matter what happens to that proposal, no matter how radically it will have to change before the United States can pass a comprehensive and realistic health-reform law, Matthew, Ebony, and Aaron were born at the moment when Americans decided that basic, decent health care should be a right. It never was before. These vulnerable children, these new citizens, were given a promise that their political leaders must now try to find a way to keep.

3

CONDITION: CRITICAL

THE children born at the Kaiser hospital in Walnut Creek had their first encounter with American medicine in one of the more reliable and reasonably priced parts of this nation's vast health-care system. Wait until they see the rest of America's medical machine. While they are still in diapers, the rest of us are busily mortgaging their future, heedlessly turning open the tap of America's wealth in a medical economy that, for all of its remarkable achievements, often seems to bear no relation to common sense when it comes to prices, allocation of resources, response to consumer demand, or even, at times, results.

Every morning, 827,000 Americans wake up in a hospital bed.[1] By the end of the day, they and their fellow citizens have spent more than $2.7 billion for medical care. That comes to $113 million every hour, $31,500 every second. Americans pay their 650,000 doctors about $540 million per day, for an average of $830 apiece. The 6,634 hospitals get more than $1 billion a day. Nursing homes take in about $218 million a day, and counting.[2] All together, the United States devoted 14 percent of its wealth to medical

27

care in 1993, nearly half again the share of GDP that most industrialized nations spent on health services. Only thirty years ago, the U.S. health bill added up to just 6 percent of the gross domestic product. But at the rate that health costs are now growing, the United States will be spending one-third of all of its resources on medicine within about twenty-five years. Theoretically, without substantial intervention in the way the system works, that level would reach more than three-fourths of all U.S. resources by the year 2050. "Health-care costs have created an American state of siege," says Florida governor Lawton Chiles. "If we don't do something about them right now, we won't have enough left over for education and transportation and all of the other things we need."[3]

In the absence of meaningful health-care reform, Americans will drive their standard of living ever lower, paying extravagantly for health services through higher taxes, lower salaries, declining productivity, job losses, and business failures. And for what? For all that we are spending, we are not that much healthier — or sicker — than other nations. United States health spending is so high mainly because of the wasteful way in which we pay for medical services. The U.S. health machine employs about fifteen million Americans[4] and constantly adds more jobs, in bad economic times as well as good. It bristles with too many specialists, too much surgery, too many accountants and clerks and personal-injury lawyers. It has an excess of hospital beds, high-tech machines, and testing laboratories. Until now, though, most medical care has not been held accountable for its value or its cost. Studies by the Rand Corporation suggest that one-fourth of all medical spending may be unnecessary. Yet it often seems that no one is watching the cash register. The challenge of health reform is to find a way to spend the money more intelligently, to find out what sort of medicine we really need, and then to maintain the quality of medical care while controlling overall costs.

No one has been able to do it so far. Already, U.S. health-care costs are so high that approximately 15 percent of Americans — an estimated 38.9 million people — are thought to be uninsured.[5] Millions cannot afford to see a doctor or to pay the hospital in case of an emergency. Worse, even as the medical bills spiral out of control, the doctors are becoming inaccessible in remote rural areas and in the devastated hearts of our cities. In some of the wealthiest cities in the world, illnesses like tuberculosis and measles are making a comeback. Meanwhile, about 17 percent of all Americans suffering from diabetes and high blood pressure are going without treatment.[6] Many of them will needlessly end up in emergency rooms, if they don't die first. A 1989 study found that up to half of all inner-city hospitalizations for the uninsured involved conditions that could easily have been treated by a family doctor or prevented altogether. Instead of finding a way to treat those patients in the early stages of their illnesses, we end up paying for life saving intervention after their diseases worsen. It is not that we lack medical resources, but that many people cannot seem to get to them. Meanwhile, the rest often get more medicine than they need. During any given year, just 1 percent of the U.S. population accounts for an astonishing 29 percent of all medical costs, while 5 percent, mainly elderly and severely injured, dying patients, generate half of the total bill.[7]

Something is wrong with the way we are spending all of this money. In a sense, the United States is beginning to resemble a lost land from *Gulliver's Travels,* a strange realm of relatively affluent and healthy people who obsessively tinker with their bodies, constantly seeking medical services even while pointing with horror at those around them who cannot afford the same care.

*   *   *

Consider the following simple facts:

• Americans devote enormous resources to fighting
off death and battling the final stages of disease. Nearly
one-third of all U.S. health-care costs — a total of about
$300 billion each year [8] — are incurred treating people
who are in the last six months of their lives. Those
patients include the people struck by catastrophic injury
and illness and millions of elderly Americans who will
die despite the heroic efforts of their physicians.

• Similarly, 35 percent of Medicare spending, or
about $45 billion, is spent on so-called futile care, a
reference to medical help that cannot possibly save patients or significantly extend their lives. "My mother
was dying of cancer," recalls one Californian, "and
they wanted to take off her leg. She asked me what I
thought. I told her to go home and be with Dad. She
didn't have much time." Clearly, much of the sort of
futile treatment that this man's mother rejected is
pointless as well as unnecessarily painful for the patients, who might otherwise die more peacefully. Dr.
James Todd, executive vice president of the American
Medical Association, agrees. He says: "We are still living in a can-do medical environment; if there is a procedure available, we give it. That has to change."[9] But
where do we cross the line between prolonging life
and prolonging death?

By focusing so many of our efforts on interfering
with the conditions that end life, we are harder
pressed to find the resources for the maintenance of
health. This unbalanced system is teetering ever more
precariously as the population ages. Through taxes,
working Americans pay most of the costs of the extensive medical treatment needed by the elderly. Their

burden is growing. There are now about seven Americans under the age of sixty-five for every person past that age.[10] That ratio has narrowed from eleven to one in 1960, and it continues to shrink. Of those seven Americans, one is unemployed and two are children. That leaves four workers to support the benefits of each older American. One of those workers is uninsured.

When the Medicare program began in 1966, it was seen as a modest program to help protect elderly Americans on fixed incomes, but the entitlement did not take personal income into account. As a result, millionaires, some of them with the most lustrous names in American business and politics, get the same subsidized care as do the elderly poor. Medicare spending is expected to exceed $200 billion by the end of this decade. It is time to ask people to pay their fair share. But no one likes to cut entitlements that they can look forward to collecting themselves. And no one in Washington seems to have the courage to face down the powerful elderly lobby. Yet.

• All in all, Americans will spend more than $1 trillion on medical care in 1994, nearly four times what they spent in 1980. By the end of this decade, the medical bill is expected to pass $1.5 trillion. That means that, by then, nearly one out of every five dollars will be spent on health care.

• Doctors admit that they probably waste anywhere from $15 billion to $100 billion every year on unnecessary medical procedures. No one knows the extent of the waste. Some physicians are not sure which tests and treatments will work best; there are new ones coming along all the time, and it takes a while to learn each one. In addition, many physicians have a financial incentive to order up a test or administer a treatment, particularly if they own a piece of the testing lab or are paid a separate fee for every procedure they perform. Moreover, many doctors are pressured by patients who really think they need an MRI or some other test they just read about in a consumer magazine. Dramatic reports of new diagnostic tests always lead to surges in patient demand, whether or not the tests are needed. Doctors call the phenomenon "the disease du jour."

Finally, doctors engage in a wasteful practice called defensive medicine to protect themselves against the constant threat and onerous costs of malpractice. In a 1992 study, eight out of ten doctors told the American Medical Association that they had ordered up extra tests for fear of being sued if they missed something. How much do defensive medicine and other wasteful practices add to U.S. health-care costs? No one knows for sure. One guesstimate (the figure that President Clinton cited in his September 1993 address to Congress) placed this total share of waste, including unnecessary procedures of all kinds, as high as $200 billion. Whatever the total, everyone knows it is very large. Many researchers are trying to learn enough to trim the waste without hurting quality. One study underway at Kaiser is examining a simple blood test administered to newborn babies. Kaiser found that only one abnormal result was found for every 750 normal tests. While any hospital would want to discover that one abnormal reading, Kaiser doctors reason that it must be possible to eliminate some of the other 750 tests. They are now trying to fine-tune their knowledge and get that ratio down to 250 to 1.[11]

• Medical prices of all kinds rise like untended hot-air balloons, seeming to float free from the laws of supply and demand. The bill for the same operation can be $21,000 or $84,000 at hospitals within a hundred-mile radius, but which doctors are the best? They're not all the same, and you can't tell by the prices. A prospective heart patient sorting through the information available to her is hard-pressed to make an intelligent selection of the most important doctor she has ever needed.

Elsewhere on the medical bill, an aspirin, given in a hospital, can cost nothing or $1.00 or $3.50 or $5.00. Same aspirin. Other costs simply seem unbelievable, as if someone had accidentally added a few zeroes. Bone-marrow transplants cost $150,000 or more. Even when a patient does not need surgery, a few days in the hospital can add up to $15,000. A couple of weeks of hospital treatment for a stroke victim can bring in bills for $50,000. Attempting to put medical costs in perspective, *Fortune* magazine surveyed companies with good benefits plans to find out how much business they had to do to pay for a standard appendectomy for an employee. Dayton Hudson reported that it must sell 39,000 Ninja Turtles; Atlantic Richfield figured it had to sell 192,000 gallons of gas, while Goodyear said it must sell 461 radial tires.[12] The analogies may be amusing, but still the numbers do not make sense.

• We spend close to $100 billion per year on medical paperwork alone, according to a Harvard study, filling out incomprehensible forms for Medicare, Medicaid, and some fifteen hundred different insurance companies with different rules. Hospitals devote entire floors to the files, and providers hire four times as many clerks as medical professionals to keep up with the paper. Private insurers alone are not to blame. The Medicare and Medicaid systems are strangling in paperwork, thanks to some 300,000 pages of federal rules.[13] No physician can possibly understand or remember all of the rules. No one can justify the paper costs.

And yet:

What are we getting for all this money?

• About one in nine American working families has no health insurance, according to rough federal estimates. Many of these people say they are neither poor enough for Medicaid nor rich enough to afford their own insurance. According to recent studies, though, about a fourth of these Americans can afford insurance but would rather skip the cost. One two-income family that made $80,000 in 1992 explained that insurance was just too expensive.[14] In general, all of these people are treated when they really need care in hospital emergency rooms, at much higher cost than if they had seen a private physician. When the uninsured receive such care, whether or not they could have afforded insurance, everyone else picks up the cost in the form of higher taxes, as well as higher insurance premiums and medical prices. In 1991, hospitals provided $13.4 billion in unpaid care.[15] Local governments (translation: taxpayers) picked up $2.6 billion of that burden through special appropriations. The rest was buried in the bills of insured patients. That's not all. Including so-called undercompensated care, such as the treatment delivered under Medicaid and Medicare price controls that are lower than actual

hospital costs, this form of cost-shifting in hospitals to-
tals about $22 billion per year.[16]

• One in three American workers has a part-time,
temporary, or project job, and their ranks are growing
rapidly. By the end of this decade, Clinton's secretary
of labor Robert Reich expects that only about half of
America's workers will have an old-fashioned, permanent job with benefits. Most of the rest are doing without benefits, or with only tenuous, temporary, or
partial coverage. And because these workers have no
long-term financial stability, many of them are finding
it impossible to afford private health insurance and are
skimping on normal preventive care, thereby risking
undetected illnesses.

• About 10 million American children are growing
up without regular checkups by doctors and dentists.[17]
Most of their parents have jobs. Unexamined by doctors, some of these children are developing chronic or
crippling illnesses that medicine learned to treat long
ago. These children are locked out of American medicine's miraculous realm. Their impaired health will
make them less-productive workers. And who will
blame these young Americans when they grow up if
they object to shouldering the fast-growing burden of
providing medical entitlements to their elders?

• Whatever happened to the family doctor? The
United States has twice as many doctors now as it did
twenty years ago,[18] but fewer and fewer Americans
can find a family doctor when they need one. Many
health experts think that in order to provide a good
balance between preventive care and more complex
medicine, about half of all doctors should be family

practitioners. But right now, nearly three-fourths are specialists who do not treat the full range of family medical needs. Worse, only about one in six medical students graduating in 1992 planned to become a general practitioner,[19] and only one in twelve students still in medical school was planning to do so.[20]

Even if medical schools started graduating nothing but family physicians tomorrow — a disastrous course that would soon wipe out needed skills and devastate medical quality as older specialists retired — it would take ten years before these family doctors added up to half of the physicians in practice. If half of all new doctors became generalists starting tomorrow, it would take fifty years before half of American physicians were generalists.[21] Asks one doctor: "Do you think the American people are going to stand for that?"

Educating substantially more family doctors is critical. But the only way to adequately relieve the shortage of family physicians is for a significant number of specialists to switch to family practice. Before they can do the job as family doctors, many of these highly trained physicians are going to need to learn new skills, such as how to treat the problems of infants and children, women, or older patients. Convincing them that they should do so is another issue: given a choice, most specialists would rather not practice as generalists.[22]

• General Motors lost $23.5 billion in 1992. That was by far the largest corporate loss in U.S. history and was triggered when GM accounted for the first time for its outstanding obligations to pay for retiree medical care.[23] Several other giant corporations followed suit with startling losses attributed to the same costs, which formerly had not been carried on their balance sheets as continuing obligations. In fact, the collective 1992 profits for all of the Fortune 500 companies totaled just $10.5 million. If they had not carried the retiree costs on their balance sheets, these companies would have reported profits of $70.5 billion.[24] Like other old-line manufacturing firms that have offered generous benefits for many years, GM is now having trouble keeping all of the promises it has made. The company provides health benefits to twice as many retirees as active workers. All in all, GM spends more on medical costs than on steel, adding nearly $1,400 to the price of every car.[25]

Facing more than $1 trillion in obligations for retiree benefits alone, a growing number of American companies are doing what they swore right through the late 1980s they would never do: dumping their retiree health plans. Elderly Americans who finished their working lives secure in the knowledge that they had earned solid pensions and superior medical coverage now regularly receive letters from their old employers abruptly canceling the promises. At least the retirees can turn to Medicare. The companies that have not canceled the plans, though, still have those bills to pay. Something's got to give.

• The fastest-growing industry in the United States is the HMO business. About 45 million Americans now receive their medical care through these health maintenance organizations, which focus heavily on family practice and specialize in holding down costs.[26] A survey of major employers by the Towers Perrin consulting firm found that companies paid 12 percent more in 1993 than they did in 1992 for employee medical coverage under traditional indemnity plans, while the costs for HMO coverage rose just 9 percent. The gap is growing. In 1994, while indemnity insurers say they will again raise their prices by about 12 percent, HMOs expect to raise their prices by only 5.6 percent on average.[27] Despite their lower costs, HMOs often enjoy spectacular profits. Example: United HealthCare, a Minnesota-based firm that manages health services for nearly 23 million Americans, reported revenues of $1.4 billion in 1992, up 70 percent from 1991, and record profits of $114 million, a 53 percent increase over the prior year.[28] The price performance of HMOs, along with their robust profits, suggests that there is still plenty of room for savings in a more competitive marketplace as more Americans join such programs and employers learn to bargain harder.

• As much as $75 billion in health spending is lost every year to outright theft and fraud.[29] When one of the largest insurance companies surveyed its customers, two out of five patients said they knew that their doctors had cheated insurance companies, generally by exaggerating their medical problems in order to qualify for higher reimbursement.[30] In many cases, of course, the patients went along with it — or even encouraged it — to make sure that their share of the costs was fully reimbursed. A patient who visits the doctor with a bad cold, for example, might not be reimbursed; but if the doctor calls the problem "gastroenteritis" (stomach flu), both doctor and patient will benefit when the insurer pays. And that's just the small stuff, even though it does add up.

The Medicaid program is a sitting duck for theft. Every year, Medicaid pays billions in fraudulent insurance claims. In 1991, California officials uncovered a spectacular scam, a $1 billion Medicaid rip-off. It was carried out by con artists operating mobile clinics in vans that cruised neighborhoods offering meaningless free medical tests. By doing so, they obtained everyone's insurance identification, then sent in countless phony claims for all sorts of medical services before being caught. In most inner cities, fly-by-night Medicaid mills offer atrocious medical service or none at all, gaming the poorly administered system like a cash cow. Often, the mills are a front for narcotics dealing or black-market drug rings. In some mills, Medicaid patients are given prescriptions, which they then sell to operatives waiting outside, collecting a small profit. The operatives resell the legal drugs to crooked pharmacies nearby, which then sell them again to the Medicaid mills. In this way, the mills can collect federal reimbursement many times for the same bottle of pills, which none of the "patients" needed in the first place. The thieves move on when state officials take notice.[31]

The American way of health is fraught with contradictions, every miracle seemingly matched by a tale of outrage or heartbreak. During the past century, American medical science has evolved all the way from patent medicine and quacks to MRI scanners, microsurgery, and the looming field of gene therapy. It has harnessed the body's natural defenses with antibiotics and other medications, has conquered plagues and diseases, and has learned how to make spare parts for almost every organ except the brain. People live longer. Crippling diseases no longer have to mean constricted lives in a relative's spare bedroom. Along the way, U.S. medical technology, drugs, and surgical skills have become the envy of other nations. Americans no longer view medicine simply in terms of seeking its intervention when they are in big trouble. Our expectations are much higher

now: we expect medicine to eliminate our physical problems and to hold off the ravages of age. We demand these
things from medicine because so often it can deliver them.

There is no doubt about it: American medicine is the best
in the world — if you can afford it.

And why does it all cost so much? Says one Californian,
an early retiree who is startled by the rising costs of his medical care at a time in his life when his medical needs are
growing: "When did we decide as a nation that every doctor
is entitled to a BMW or two?" The resentment continues to
grow. Those with coverage are afraid that it is only a matter
of time before they join the ranks of the uninsured, and
they blame doctors, hospitals, and insurance companies. In
a *Time*/CNN poll conducted by Yankelovich, 91 percent of
those surveyed said that "our health-care system needs fundamental change." What kind? In the survey, 83 percent
said they'd start by cutting doctors' fees.[32] The United States
has now embarked on an effort to fix what's wrong with its
health-care structure. What kinds of changes are made, and
at what cost, and who will pay, and what we will be willing
to give up in the process, will be the central questions of the
health-policy debate that will unfold in the year to come.

When President Clinton gave his rousing and eloquent
speech in favor of health system reform before a joint session of Congress on September 22, 1993, he emphasized six
guiding principles upon which he said he based his ideas for
reform:

> Security, Simplicity, Savings, Choice, Quality, and Re-
> sponsibility.
>
> We can no longer afford to continue to ignore what is
> wrong. Millions of Americans are just a pink slip away
> from losing their health insurance, and one serious ill-
> ness away from losing all their savings. Millions more are
> locked into the jobs they have now just because they or

someone in their family has once been sick and they have what is called a preexisting condition. And on any given day, over 37 million Americans, most of them working people and their little children, have no health insurance at all. And in spite of all this, our medical bills are growing at over twice the rate of inflation and the United States spends over a third more of its income on health care than any other nation on Earth, and the gap is growing, causing many of our companies in global competition severe disadvantage. There is no excuse for this kind of system.

Everyone seems to agree that certain broad reforms are necessary. As President Clinton put it that night: "For the first time in this century, leaders of both political parties have joined together around the principle of providing universal comprehensive health care. It is a magic moment, and we must seize it."

Even more important, it is not just the political leaders who have come together on the basic principles of reform. Not only conservative Republicans and liberal Democrats support reform, but also the American Medical Association and other physician groups, the American Hospital Association, the Pharmaceutical Manufacturers Association, the Health Insurance Association of America, the U.S. Chamber of Commerce, and other business groups and health providers. Moreover, the consensus is about more than finding a way to provide basic health care to all Americans. Just about everyone also agrees that continuity of care should be ensured through insurance reform. The Health Insurance Association of America represents the firms that write 70 percent of all U.S. commercial coverage,[33] including such giants as Mutual of Omaha and John Hancock. The Health Insurance Association of America has maintained for some time that companies must eliminate the practice of dropping people when they get sick or when it is discovered that they have chronic conditions or are at risk for complicated diseases. Finally, everyone, it seems, now sees that national health spending must somehow be brought under control and made more equitable.

The agenda for health reform now facing Americans is daunting. Its two principal goals — expanding coverage and controlling costs — are inherently contradictory. Only a masterly legislative effort will be able to achieve both while also maintaining the quality of medical care. President Clinton deserves enormous credit for giving this program the highest political priority. Despite the efforts of many political leaders before him, no one has been able to ensure comprehensive coverage or to get the costs under control; he wants to do both. And no matter how many political leaders or medical and business groups support these goals, they disagree strongly on the means that would be acceptable to achieve them. Only wise and strong political leadership in the White House and in the Congress can forge a workable reform law. Many others have tried, and all of them have failed. As President Clinton has said, now that everyone seems committed to finding a way, it is time to seize the moment.

4

THE POLITICS OF REFORM

PRESIDENT Clinton's proposed legislation to reform the health-care system has been heralded as the most sweeping and important domestic program since the Social Security Act of 1935. If so, a special irony is worth noting. National health insurance was part of the original Social Security legislation. It was dropped, largely at the insistence of the American Medical Association. Even in 1935, the AMA worried that greater federal involvement in medicine would impinge on physician independence and result in lower quality of care.[1] Americans have been arguing over how to reform their balky and wasteful health-care system for a very long time. Babies have been born, gone to medical school, and retired while we have been debating the same questions of quality, equity, and cost.

In the years since Social Security was enacted, one political leader after another has carried the banner of national health insurance, only to see it torn to pieces. President Lyndon Johnson got the closest, seeing Medicare and Medicaid enacted in 1965, but Medicaid was in trouble within a year and remains a deeply flawed and enormously expensive mess. President Nixon tried to expand the Medicare concept to cover all Americans, but by the time he raised the issue, Watergate was pulling him under. President Bush called for comprehensive health reform, but he put that on his list of things to do in the second term that he did not win. Senator Edward Kennedy can count a gray hair for every time he has sallied forth with hearings and proposals for the cause. Year after year, countless bills aiming for substantial reform have died or have been left on base at the end of congressional sessions. Beginning in the late 1980s, the legislative momentum began to build, with flight after flight of bills arcing like arrows into the public arena, all of them falling short, each congressional session ending in the usual stasis. Beltway analysts branded health reform as one of those challenges, like dieting, that everyone seems to need to talk about, but nobody seems able to carry through. The experts said that health care was a boring, no-win issue: nobody understood it, and besides, most Americans felt pretty good about their own coverage, didn't they? Better not fool with it.

Well then, why now? How did health-care reform vault to the top of the national agenda? And what are the odds it will stay there?

The passionate national consensus for health reform is rooted in the great expectations that have come tumbling down during the past fifteen years as the U.S. economy has restructured itself. While the American economy became more dynamic as companies grew more competitive, workers suffered. Millions of them lost high-paying jobs. Many of them became mired in downward mobility and uncertainty, unable to adjust to economic changes as quickly as investment capital can. During the 1980s, the Fortune 500, the large corporations that traditionally provided the most generous benefits, cut the ranks of their workers by more than 3 million. After several years of slashing staff size, those employers then began subcontracting entire functions to outside firms, untethering even more workers from the benefits offered to those who remained on staff.

While some of these subcontractors offered pay and benefits roughly comparable to the old company plan, most workers were not so lucky. Even in the midst of the Reagan boom, when some 20 million jobs were being created, the job and health insecurity were growing. Nearly all of those jobs were being created by small businesses, the ones least able to afford good benefits. In addition, millions of the new jobs were part-time, contract, and other types of contingent work that carried no long-term security or benefits. While the new contingent employees were often happy to have fairly steady work, their pay was usually a fraction of what it had been, which made it even harder to do anything about the fact that when they lost their "good" job, they also lost their health insurance.

Most people assumed that companies were turning permanent workers into temps and part-timers mainly to save money on benefits. But the corporate disengagement from long-term relationships with workers went deeper than that. Employers admitted privately that they were not only getting out of all those expensive benefits obligations but were also escaping the broader burden of years of accumulated employee rights and implied company promises that made it harder to hire, promote, or fire workers at will. "The way business is today," said one CEO in 1993, "the last thing you want to do is make one more promise to one more worker." So they didn't. Companies added jobs much more warily than they once did. Nobody used the term "permanent" anymore to refer to workers. When employers "self-insured," setting up their own insurance for employees, they often limited coverage of expensive medical problems, refusing, for instance, to pay more than a small amount for

AIDS coverage. Everyone yearned for the old sense of security, of being part of something bigger than themselves.
Insurance was no longer something you could count on.
Said one worker, "They'd better start calling it something
else, don't you think?" Health coverage that had always
seemed free was no longer either cheap or certain. Insurance companies, seeking ways to preserve their profits and
unable to raise premiums fast enough to match pace with
rising costs, had begun to engage in once-unthinkable practices. Coverage for entire companies was canceled, sometimes when just a few employees fell expensively ill. This
was particularly true for small firms, which faced sky-high
premiums and were more vulnerable to policy cancelations
because their costs could not be spread over a large group.
Meanwhile, more and more individuals were denied insurance because of the frightening term "preexisting conditions," meaning medical problems and chronic conditions
the insurer did not care to take on. In any given year, about
30 million Americans change jobs; suddenly, many of them
found that once they did, they were unable to replace their
insurance benefits. Between 1989 and 1992 alone, 3 million
Americans lost employer coverage.[2] One family after another found itself facing the specter of illness without satis-
factory coverage, wondering what had happened to their
dreams of rising living standards and financial security. One
by one, American families had come to live in fear of illness,
of medical bills that defy any realistic prospect of payment.
Already burdened with excessive consumer debt and facing
an often-uncertain economic future, they grew more and
more enraged over medical costs.

Job insecurity had never provoked the passion that medical insecurity did. Medicine is different from other basic
needs. It is more personal than food, jobs, or housing. After
all, needing medical help is one of the most profoundly disturbing and frightening experiences anyone can have. The

helpless patient is confronted with the mystery of the malfunctioning Self and needs to be rescued by the physician. Illness without ready treatment is terrifying, especially when it has never happened to you before. The doctor is supposed to be there when things go wrong. Withholding care is unforgivable.

As the 1980s drew to a close, many of the angry and frightened Americans outraged by medical costs were middle-class workers who had never known such anxiety about the future and never expected that they would. After all, their parents had not, but their parents had raised families in a less-threatening time of steady economic expansion and insignificant foreign competition. As employers lightened their benefits load, shifting a larger share of medical costs to workers, even the well insured began to feel betrayed. Whether or not their reaction to their often insignificant new responsibility for health costs was unreasonable, these workers had come to believe that one way or another, the rules always change, and never in their favor.

Suddenly, in the fall of 1991, as the presidential campaign year was about to begin, health care became the litmus test of American politics. In Pennsylvania, an obscure Democrat named Harris Wofford handily defeated the popular former governor and U.S. attorney general Richard Thornburgh in a race for the U.S. Senate by calling for a health-care plan that would cover everyone. The leaders of both political parties were astounded by the election results. Nobody had realized that the promise of reliable health coverage could wield such political punch. An issue that had bobbed at the edge of the political mainstream for nearly sixty years, driven back again and again by apathy and the various groups opposing change, had suddenly become the make-or-break issue of politics on the eve of the presidential campaign.

Health care and Bill Clinton were a perfect fit. He ran as a populist, a small-town hero from a town called Hope who promised Change. President Bush promised health-care reform too, but his heart did not seem to be in it. He seemed hopelessly disengaged from domestic issues, unable to understand why people were upset. Bill Clinton was passionate about the issue; he promised he would drive the money-changers out of medicine's temple and make superior, reliable health care affordable for all Americans, and he promised to spell out his plan of attack within a hundred days of taking office.

Once he was elected, that deadline slipped, and another, and another, from March, to April, to May, to June, and on and on, as the administration worked on The Plan. Almost every day, it seemed, the newspapers were printing new White House versions of what would be in the proposal, as well as revised timetables for its unveiling. Since no one else seemed to be getting much attention for a health-care plan, though, and the president's staff talked incessantly about the one he was working on, health reform was becoming equated in the public mind with the president's forthcoming proposal.

Meanwhile, President Clinton mounted Stage One of his attack immediately, by putting his wife, Hillary Rodham Clinton, in charge of shaping the health-care program. It was a novel, possibly brilliant, political tactic. This unprecedented assignment for a First Lady drew enthusiastic public support and kept the spotlight on the energetic First Family commitment to reform. Congressional opponents were cowed, but only for a while.

What do most Americans want to see in a health-care reform plan? First of all, they want to see the president's signature on it, and soon. They want President Clinton to use his power to kick some sense into the medical system. Beyond that, there is much disagreement about what is wrong and how it should be fixed. In an informal survey of about three hundred interested citizens conducted during the summer and fall of 1993, this author was told by different people that the main problem with health care was drug prices, or doctors' prices, or the greed of insurance companies, or dishonest hospitals that send questionable bills, or plans that cut corners on medical treatment to save money. Some said that the most urgent need is for more family physicians; one temporary worker suggested that President Clinton could clear up the whole problem by signing an executive order immediately admitting 100,000 foreign-born family doctors to the United States, so long as they commit themselves to serving where they are needed. Many people were convinced that other countries have licked the problem of providing first-rate health care to all, though they were vague on the details. Some wondered if the health-care crisis had been invented by politicians, since they did not see it in their own lives. They worried that in trying to help those who have too little coverage, the administration will ask everyone else to pay too much and will take away their choices in health care. One way or another, many people were deeply skeptical that the federal government could fix what's broken in health care. They liked the president's appealing passion; it was the idea of new government intrusion into such a personal area that worried them. Many rejected the notion that everyone must be guaranteed the same health benefits.

The Clinton administration has assured Americans that it will deliver something that is better than what they already have. That's a tall order. Moreover, in fixing the parts of the health-care system that are not working well, the president also proposes to change the parts that people like. He wants to replace a patchwork quilt of coverage with a new, unified plan that offers everyone basically the same thing. He

believes that is the only way to get control of costs and ensure health security for everyone. Inevitably, though, such a
broad scheme for reform will make people uncomfortable.
Many people are a bit gun-shy about the changes they have
already been through, with new restrictions placed on their
employee medical coverage or on their choice of doctors.
The American way of health has evolved rapidly during
the past fifteen years, and lately the pace has been picking
up. Until recently, medical care was characterized primarily
by private relationships with independent physicians. Insurers waited to get bills, then paid them. But starting in the
mid-1970s, employers and insurance companies began to
question the decisions that individuals and doctors were
making on medical treatment. American medicine entered
a new epoch, the era of managed care.

The idea behind managed care was simple enough: those
who paid the medical bills — corporations as well as insurance companies — wanted to see that these huge amounts
of money were spent efficiently, rather than wastefully.
From the employers' point of view, health care was the only
major expense they were not managing, and the costs
seemed to be out of control. Insurers, too, thought it was
time they had something to say about the billions of dollars
they were paying out, especially since the higher the bills,
the more they had to raise premiums to cover them. These
payers asserted the right to question the way doctors went
about treating patients and to challenge surgery or tests or
extra days in the hospital that might not be necessary. Typically, in managed-care plans, a patient was required to seek
a second opinion before surgery or hospitalization. Under
managed care, everything done for a patient was supposed
to make sense. Insurance companies hired doctors and
nurses to look over the shoulders of the physicians treating
their clients; these new workers scanned the bills and picked
up the phone to ask the physicians questions. Doctors had to

defend their decisions regarding treatment if they wanted to be reimbursed. Sometimes, when the insurance company thought they had done things that were not needed, the doctors were not paid. Doctors learned to think twice before prescribing certain treatments.

As the managed-care approach grew, those providing the medical care adjusted the way they did it. Instead of each physician and hospital making decisions on the spur of the moment, organized groups of doctors began to offer new kinds of health plans that promised cost-conscious care. These plans included preventive treatment as part of their coverage, on the theory that it was worth paying to keep people healthier instead of just waiting until they got sick enough to seek treatment for serious medical problems. Health maintenance organizations (HMOs), which offered all-around medical treatment and kept track of a patient's overall health, began to enroll more people. Preferred Provider Organizations (PPOs) were also spreading; in this type of health plan model, a group of doctors would negotiate a deal with a company to cover its employees at a certain cost, usually setting their prices somewhat below average physician fees in the area.

The 1980s saw large employers beginning to wield their health buying power in an organized fashion, demanding more such volume discounts for their employee health care. Since they represented large numbers of potential patients, they could negotiate prices with hospitals, HMOs, PPOs, and other managed-care plans seeking business. At the same time, insurance companies were becoming health-care companies, branching out from simply financing medicine to providing it. They began to set up their own HMOs and PPOs and to offer other kinds of medical services. Confronting the new cost-sensitive managed-care environment, nonprofit hospitals entered the era of modern management, paying attention for the first time to cutting waste.

The last great cottage industry in America was undergoing consolidation. By the time health care became the leading domestic issue in 1993, the majority of U.S. doctors had affiliated themselves in various ways with managed-care plans.[3] Some, who remained in private practice, agreed to go along with an HMO's rules, for example, when treating those of their patients who were signed up with the plan. Those rules might stipulate second opinions before hospitalization or might limit the doctor's freedom to refer patients to specialists or to order up diagnostic testing, such as extra blood tests or X-rays. Other doctors had become employees of HMOs or had joined PPOs or other large physician groups, following the rules of the organization when they treated patients.

At the same time, large teaching hospitals were beginning to build their own diversified medical networks instead of contenting themselves with simply signing contracts to do surgery for HMOs and other health plans. These hospitals linked up with clinics and groups of doctors to offer their own value-priced, comprehensive health coverage. The Mayo Clinic affiliated itself with groups of doctors throughout the Midwest, offering them clinical support. In Manhattan, the New York Hospital formed an integrated health network, buying up smaller area hospitals and clinics and setting up its own HMO in order to offer its own version of one-stop medical shopping to people in the extended metropolitan area. In Chicago and Los Angeles, similar networks were created. In Boston, Massachusetts General Hospital announced a plan in December of 1993 to merge with Brigham and Women's Hospital. The two teaching affiliates of the Harvard Medical School had long been fierce competitors; but together, as the state's third-largest employer, they will link up with smaller community hospitals, physician groups, and managed-care plans to provide a comprehensive health network.

One reason that hospitals are forming integrated networks is that they have become uncomfortably dependent upon managed-care plans sending them patients. By integrating vertically in the new networks, these hospitals can offer more services and perhaps better prices than competing hospitals when managed-care plans shop around. Once they add a few neighborhood clinics and outpatient centers, some of these networks are becoming the primary health plan in which patients are enrolled. Such networks will cut the HMO out of the deal, thereby ensuring themselves a steady flow of income as patients come to them directly.

As the competition to offer more cost-effective health care has been growing, so has the competition to control groups of insured patients. In medicine, patients are the key commodity, the reason that doctors and hospitals get paid. In the past, patients became customers one at a time and had little leverage in challenging prices or treatments. Medicine essentially was a seller's market. But in the new world of managed care, patients usually are found in large groups, such as the staff of an entire company that orchestrates coverage for its employees or the membership of an HMO that decides which hospitals and doctors can serve its patients.

More and more, medicine is becoming a buyer's market. Those who provide medical care must work harder to attract significant numbers of patients. When Americans go to specialists these days, they are often taken aback when the specialists eagerly tell them, "I can be your primary doctor too." Why is the specialist suddenly so interested in practicing general medicine? Because in managed care, it is the primary care doctor who is assured of a steady stream of revenue, not the specialist. The primary care doctor always sees the patient first, then decides whether the patient needs to see a specialist. And what is a primary care doctor? Dr. William Rodney, chairman of the Department of Family Medicine at the University of Tennessee, Memphis, says with a chuckle, "He's the first guy who gets to you when you need help, and the race is on!"

It is, indeed. In some places, doctors are fighting fiercely over the right to serve patients. During the summer of 1993, two specialist groups, the American Society for Gastrointestinal Endoscopy and the American College of Gastroenterology, jointly launched a major offensive against family physicians across the United States. The gastroenterologists were determined to stop family doctors from performing endoscopy, a type of test in which a doctor examines a patient's colon or upper gastrointestinal tract; these tests are used to check for colon cancer and other problems. The price is usually at least a couple of hundred dollars, depending on the nature of the examination. The two groups of specialists hired Williams and Connolly, a big-league Washington law firm, to make their case that family doctors were not adequately trained to perform these procedures. The lawyers rendered an opinion that since the specialists who had retained them were so much more skilled at the tests, any hospital allowing family doctors to come in and perform such a test on a patient was in dire danger of a major malpractice suit.

This information was sent to hospitals all over the United States. Hospitals began barring family doctors from performing the tests. Says Dr. Rodney, a lifelong family physician: "They did not want family doctors taking away their business. But family doctors practice in a lot of small towns where there are no specialists, and hospitals in some of those towns are now barring family doctors from doing this. The public-health tragedy is that these procedures prevent premature deaths from colorectal cancer. Therefore, to prevent the widespread use of these procedures is tantamount to the development of an economic cartel at the expense of the American public. This is particularly tragic for rural and underserved communities, where the best chance to receive these preventive care services is from a family physician."[4]

By the fall of 1993, as President Clinton prepared to introduce his health-reform plan, American medicine had already moved deep into managed-care territory. Patients were getting out of hospitals sooner; many were being treated on an outpatient basis instead. Some medical costs were dropping dramatically. In Florida, Columbia / HCA Healthcare, the largest U.S. hospital chain, offered a local health purchasing cooperative a 40 percent discount off normal costs to win its medical business and barely nailed the contract in spirited bidding.[5] Across the country, doctors were comparing notes and, in some cases, deciding against surgery. Patients considering optional surgery were being shown videos in which patients like themselves explained the pluses and minuses, so that they could make informed decisions. Was it really worth it? They could decide. Every year, meanwhile, fifty obsolete and underused hospitals were closing down. Families were beginning to get used to managed care. Many preferred it. It was simpler and more convenient.

National health reform must be crafted with caution. Its guiding principle should be borrowed from medicine: Do No Harm. The White House has insisted that it will not be that difficult to fix up the trillion-dollar U.S. health-care system. The administration wants to build on the existing principle of voluntary employer-provided health insurance, making it mandatory for employers, and to put more financial discipline into health costs. By cutting out the waste, the fraud, and what they believe to be excessive drug company and insurance profits, White House officials say that not only can they offer everyone comprehensive, affordable insurance without any new broad-based taxes, but they can

also significantly cut the national deficit. They say that
Americans will like their new health-care system. They insist that Americans will have more choice. They have said
that only about 15 percent of Americans will pay more for
their coverage. That group comprises predominantly younger and healthier people. Most Americans, according to the
White House, will pay about the same for their coverage as
they now do, or in some cases, less. Finally, the administration maintains that as a result of all of these changes, everyone will have higher-quality medical care.

Is it really possible to offer everyone more, and pay less?
Can medical treatment be managed that closely without
leading providers to cut too many corners on care in order
to save money? When NBC news anchor Tom Brokaw
asked President Clinton during a November 1993 interview
whether it was true that the changes he was proposing
might bring about new rationing of medical services, the
president paused for a moment. Then he answered by saying simply that we already have rationing in the United
States.

That is true. People who do not have insurance coverage,
or doctors nearby, face rationing by default when they cannot get health care that they need. Underfunded public hospitals, as well, do not always have the resources to give poor
patients everything they need and thus are forced to ration
what they do have.

But in easing the extent of those shortages for the minority who are underserved, will the Clinton plan inflict more
of the pain of rationing on all Americans? That was the burden of Brokaw's question. By answering the question so
obliquely, the president passed up an opportunity to say it
was not true. The question remains on the table.

5

JACKSON WHO?

I've been under attack as some kind of traitor to
medicine for years. Anybody who tries to change
something about medicine is some kind of commu-
nist, a radical, and is viewed as nothing short of immoral by many doctors.
— PAUL M. ELLWOOD, M.D., August 1993

AT 5:30 one chilly August morning in 1993, the coyotes
were howling in the foothills of the Grand Tetons. A mile
up on a ridge, a light was on in a window, where Dr. Paul
Ellwood was turning on the coffee for the crowd that would
begin arriving any time now. One by one, several political leaders and some of the most powerful buyers and
providers of medical care in the country began to arrive in
his Jackson Hole, Wyoming, kitchen from their rented ski
condos farther down the mountain. The governors of Florida, Vermont, and Utah had come up from the National
Governors Association meeting in Tulsa, Oklahoma. Also
here were top executives of Blue Cross/Blue Shield and
other insurers representing 125 million Americans; the
chief executives of the Mayo Clinic, the Glaxo and Pfizer
pharmaceutical firms, and Columbia / HCA Healthcare, the
largest U.S. hospital chain; executives of General Motors and

General Electric, the American Medical Association, the
U.S. Healthcare HMO chain, and several other medical providers. Alan Greenspan, the chairman of the Federal Reserve Board, was meeting a few miles up the road with the
bankers who run the financial system, but hardly anybody
knew they were in town. It was a measure of the political
moment that plenty of people from Washington to Wyoming were curious about the deliberations of this group, the
powers in American health care. Only a couple of weeks
remained before President Clinton would unveil his health-
reform proposal before a joint session of Congress. The
Jackson Hole Group, an informal health think tank that had
contributed many of the ideas in the president's plan, was
here to discuss the emerging proposal with their political
guests.

Founded by Dr. Ellwood, the Jackson Hole Group meets
several times a year in his living room to exchange ideas
about how to improve health-care services. This time,
though, there was a tangible sense of urgency in the room.
Little by little, the Jackson Group's ideas have taken root in
Washington, D.C., and in state capitals around the country.
For that reason, some of those here had strong feelings about
the direction the president was taking with reform. Utah
governor Mike Leavitt, for one, was skeptical that Congress
would pass what he called "the mother of all unfunded federal mandates" in 1994. Others took the somewhat patron-
izing attitude that the president of the United States de-
served an A for effort, but only a C+ for execution. Why was
he adding all of these troublesome changes to the Jackson
Hole model? Why didn't he listen to them? After all, they
knew plenty about how to provide medical care. In addition,
of course, they harbored another concern: the reform effort
the president had launched would inevitably hurt some of
them, while creating immense profits for others.

*   *   *

The meeting got under way promptly at 7:30, when Ellwood, who helped launch the HMO business in the 1970s, stepped to the corner of the hearth and banged an Old West–style dinner iron. The living room where these discussions take place is imposing. Six monumental spruce trunks form the pillars of the room, standing thirty feet high and angling out from the front door toward the sunken area surrounding the fireplace. These two-hundred-year-old trees were harvested after the Yellowstone fire of 1988, and they show the scars: narrow vertical slashes where the heat popped them open, and black circles where branches once grew. The Tetons can be seen through walls of glass to either side. Above the fireplace, a mosaic of aqua stones cascades down an undulating wall like rushing water. This morning, blinding shards of sunlight were slicing across the room, which is why some of those finding seats on the sofas or on the carpeted stairs leading down toward the hearth were wearing sunglasses. For those in the harshest glare, Ellwood passed out baseball caps to help block the light. The group was dressed casually, in western shirts, Polo sweaters, jeans and chinos, hiking and cowboy boots. As they were settling down, Democratic senator Jay Rockefeller of West Virginia strolled in with his wife, Sharon, from the huge Rockefeller place down the road, about the same time Republican senator Kit Bond of Missouri clattered downstairs from a guest room.

Ellwood has been hosting these gatherings since 1970, first at his vacation condo here, then later in this home, once he moved to Wyoming. The point of these meetings has always been to get people who control hundreds of billions of dollars worth of health services to sit down and debate ideas about how to do a better job, but Ellwood was anxious that morning. Earlier, he had said the stakes for health reform had never been this high: "Some of us have worked for twenty-five years, trying to get a comprehensive reform that will touch the lives of everyone in this country. But this is new territory. Nobody has ever been this close before. It's become big-league politics now, and all kinds of political motivations are confusing the issue."[1] Not to mention the business motivations, which were well represented in this room. The day before, someone had asked: "What do they do up there, anyway? Talk about how they're going to cut up the cake?"

Until now, the Jackson Hole Group had been accustomed to debating in private. But as they gathered in late 1993, the members were suddenly seeing their carefully crafted ideas taking form as national policy. Out of such a private gathering in 1991 had come the proposal for the managed-competition plan for health reform. The National Governors Association said it was the best model for national reform. Bill Clinton had endorsed it as a presidential candidate and had used many of its elements in the plan he was now devising. Ira Magaziner, Clinton's chief health policy aide, had attended the February 1993 meeting of this group.

In reshaping health markets, managed competition seeks to ensure universal access to comprehensive health care and to consolidate consumer buying power, while also stimulating competition among providers to boost quality and hold down prices. Under the managed-competition approach, the federal government would set certain basic standards for health care, defining a benefits package that all employers would be required to offer to their workers. The benefits would ensure all Americans comprehensive health coverage, with an emphasis on preventive care and early diagnosis. These benefits would be portable, which means that Americans would not lose their coverage if they lost their jobs or moved to another company. No one could be denied coverage, and no one could lose it, regardless of his or her medical problems or financial status.

To obtain these benefits, nearly everyone would join local health purchasing cooperatives (President Clinton calls them alliances). The cooperatives would act as community purchasing agents for health care, shopping around to find the health plans offering the best quality and prices in the area. Stanford economist Alain Enthoven, coauthor with Ellwood of the basic managed-competition plan, has described these co-ops as "farmers' markets of health care." In Enthoven's view, they would be large enough to lend bargaining clout to individuals and small businesses so that they could win desirable rates from health providers. No longer would families and small businesses have to fear insurance premiums so high that they could not afford coverage. The largest corporations, already some of the savviest bargainers in buying health care, would be permitted to operate their own, separate purchasing cooperatives if they wished to do so.

Medical care would be provided by competing health plans. Doctors, hospitals, HMOs, and other providers would form health groups to bid for the co-op business. After shopping around, the cooperative would offer its members a choice of plans, ranging from a low-cost, HMO type of plan to a fee-for-service plan for which people could pay somewhat more for the right to greater choice of physicians and hospitals. Consumers would then shop among the plans selected by their co-op and sign up with the one they liked best. If too few consumers chose a particular local health plan, it might be in danger of going out of business, since the local co-op would represent just about everyone in the area. That threat would make all providers work harder to offer people the right combination of price, quality, and satisfaction. Unless they were in one of the plans chosen by the co-op, doctors and hospitals would not be able to collect insurance reimbursement for treating people who belonged to the co-op.

Corporate employee benefits would no longer be completely tax free. (Taxpayers currently spend about $50 billion per year to subsidize the employer costs of providing benefits.) Instead, companies would only write off the costs of the standard benefits package. If they chose to offer their employees benefits that were better than the standard package available to others — which they might well do as hiring incentives — the employees would pay income tax on the surplus value of the benefits. Examples of such taxable benefits might be additional dental or mental health coverage or reimbursement for eyeglasses. These changes would end tax subsidies that encourage the use of more expensive health benefits and shield companies as well as workers from the costs. All in all, the plan is designed to make patients more cost conscious while also instigating brisk competition among doctors and other providers to do a better job.

To ensure that consumers could accurately judge the quality of the care provided, all health plans would be required to provide information to the co-ops about patient satisfaction and the results of their medical treatment. The plans would report such things as the immunization rate of children they served, the quality of their prenatal care, and the success rate of their surgeons, as well as feedback from surveys of patients on how they were treated and how they fared as a result. This information would be summarized for consumers on report cards. People who suffered from lower back pain could see how a particular health plan scored in that area. People with small children could see how similar families enrolled in a plan evaluated its services. Jackson Hole called these provider groups accountable health plans, because for the first time, such standard data would hold doctors and others plainly accountable for their work. More important in the long run, it would enable health researchers, working with physicians, to study ways of improving medical care while eliminating waste. If researchers are right that anywhere from a fifth to half of all American medical treatment is of uncertain value, such research would help eliminate the unnecessary treatments and throw light on smart medical practices worth emulating.

Most of the hundred or so members of the Jackson Hole Group endorsed all of these ideas. During the last few years, virtually all of the major players in health care, from the American Medical Association and the Pharmaceutical Manufacturers Association to the major insurance companies, have called for such guarantees as universal coverage, comprehensive benefits, and portability of coverage. The members of the Jackson Hole Group are also prepared to be held publicly accountable for the quality of their work and are willing to compete in the open market for the right to serve the health needs of Americans.

The American Medical Association is still holding back from a wholehearted endorsement of the managed-competition proposal, though it participates in the meetings and applauds most of the plan. AMA leaders remain anxious about some aspects of the approach, since it limits physician independence by forcing doctors to scramble along with everyone else to please patients. Critics say the AMA is just trying to protect physician incomes. But what the AMA says is that managed competition might interfere with medical judgments about what a patient needs — and if the local rules turn out to be too restrictive, they will be proved right. Dr. James Todd, the AMA's executive vice president, says of the proposal, "Sounds like controlled competition to me. No choice for the provider."

The AMA's reservations do not prevent it from supporting Jackson Hole. Often portrayed as an uncommunicative monolith of medical power, the AMA is trying to work with other health providers toward useful reform that preserves medical quality. The members of Jackson Hole cherish the fact that they can disagree in these private meetings and try to hash out their differences. After twenty years of conversations in Ellwood's living rooms, they have formed a rough consensus behind the managed-competition proposal. Those who may still disagree with parts of the plan keep coming to Jackson Hole to argue their points and to persuade the others to compromise a bit. Ellwood explains: "We have an agreement here that we are all responsible for improving the quality of medical care and making it more affordable for everyone. They're all pushing each other forward." If so, that is an impressive achievement.

Senators Rockefeller and Bond had come to Jackson Hole to talk about their parties' clashing reform ideas. Months earlier, the Republican Senate leadership had embraced universal coverage and most of the president's other goals for reform, but Bond objected to Clinton's plan to finance it by requiring all employers to pay for comprehensive health insurance. He said that would cost too many jobs, that small business could not afford it. What was the point of giving people health insurance, he said, if it meant that they lost their jobs? Rockefeller was in no mood for compromise. He brusquely admonished those in the room who disagreed with parts of the president's plan, calling them "purists" and, later, "malcontents." He scolded Ellwood for writing an article for the *Wall Street Journal* criticizing the regulatory aspects of the plan. Rockefeller maintained that there was no time for broad debate about the reform proposal, saying that anyone in Congress who impeded Clinton's aim to pass his legislation in 1994 would be unlikely to win reelection. Bond flushed. He told Rockefeller that the Republicans were eager to work with the president on health-reform legislation and that finishing up by late 1994 sounded just fine, but he warned, "If what you want is a partisan shootout, we'll be there." Soon after this exchange, Rockefeller left the meeting. Bond stuck around to listen to the rest of the discussion.

Most sessions at Jackson Hole are a bit more subdued than the exchange of fireworks that marked the Rockefeller-Bond debate. But disagreements are common and are not always resolved. The main advantage of gathering together influential representatives from all the major sectors in health care is that ideas from anyone in the group can be tested against some of the toughest minds in the market. A typical session finds a proponent of a new idea defending it in blunt discussion with others who may have conflicting interests. At the August meeting, for example, Florida governor Lawton Chiles challenged Rick Scott, the chief executive of Columbia / HCA Healthcare. Florida had recently put its own managed-competition system into place. Nearly everyone in the state lives within twenty minutes of Columbia's forty-seven Florida hospitals. But so far, Columbia had not agreed to provide data for standard measures of accountability. Chiles wanted Scott to help Florida take reform a step further by pledging himself to begin collecting and reporting so-called outcomes information on the results of medical treatment. Scott responded crisply that he would be happy to gather such information as soon as "the market" (other hospitals and health providers) was willing to do it. In the room were executives representing dozens of other hospitals, some of which compete with Scott's, and also the top officials of the insurers that cover half of all Americans and provide direct medical services through HMOs and other managed-care plans. They, too, would be expected to report such data under the Jackson Hole model. No one volunteered; they waited for Scott to take the lead. After a tense moment, he excused himself and went out to the kitchen for a while. By the time he returned, the discussion had moved on to other points. But Scott, who was attending his first meeting, had been served notice that those who come to Jackson Hole are expected to participate in reform.

Chiles was throwing down the gauntlet because he does not feel that he can afford to wait for national reform. Accountability, after all, is a test of value, a way to make sure that low-cost providers really are doing a good job for less. Chiles said he can't wait the five or more years that it would take to get a national managed-competiton system up and running. That is why he is so determined to move ahead with Florida's system and be sure that it is working properly. "When I went to the National Governors Association meeting two years ago," he recalled, "everyone was talking about passing national reform by the year 2000. Well, I started hollering! I told them that Florida would be broke long before then. We need effective reform immediately."

Another dispute arose when Dr. Nancy Dickey, a Richmond, Texas, family physician who serves on the AMA board of trustees, insisted that in any national reform, every doctor must be allowed the right to participate in every health plan. She called the idea, which had been endorsed by the AMA, the "all willing providers" provision; she argued that it helps patients to know for sure that their doctors can join their plans. Several states have already passed laws requiring managed-care plans to allow physicians to participate if they want to. Under the co-op structure of managed competition, such a rule would mean that physicians could simply sign up with whichever health plans were popular with people in the co-op and could participate in all of them, from the low-cost version to the higher-cost plan. But at Jackson Hole, Dr. Dickey got a cold reception. One insurance executive bluntly told her that the demand had nothing to do with helping patients; face it, he said, it was only about maximizing physician incomes. Other participants compared the idea to the position of a worker who demands the right to go to any company in the country and claim a job. "Just because you are willing to work for Chrysler," said a hospital administrator, "doesn't mean that Chrysler should be forced to hire you. It doesn't make sense. You have to allow health plans to figure out how many doctors they need and pick the good ones, or else they won't be able to control their costs or compete." Though Dr. Dickey insisted that doctors were only asking for "a level playing field" so they would not be unfairly shut out of local health markets, her argument did not convince the group. Physicians, they maintained, should have to compete along with everyone else for the right to serve patients.

Ellwood generally keeps a low profile during these exchanges, encouraging the others to say what they think. Jackson Hole is first and foremost a clearinghouse for ideas from around the country. Membership is fluid: about a hundred health executives, economists, academics, and public officials have attended several times, but only ten or so have been there frequently. Depending upon the topics on the agenda, Ellwood invites experts in those areas to participate in particular meetings. But whenever the discussion drifts or bogs down, he pokes it along quietly, often with a question. There is, after all, a point to these meetings. He is trying to combine — provoke, if necessary — the best thinking of leaders in different arenas of health care in order to come up with workable ideas. He tries to guide the meetings so that, over the ebb and flow of three days, grievances are aired, problems are brought to light, and differences are accommodated. If all goes well, the sessions build to rough consensus before everyone leaves for the airport. If the group reaches unanimity on a key issue, someone on his staff of six to eight medical analysts will prepare a position paper on the issue, circulate it among the participants for comment and revisions, then distribute it on Capitol Hill and among other health experts.

That is what happened when Dr. Alan Nelson, executive vice president of the American Society of Internal Medicine, raised a point of his own. Nelson noted that the latest version of the Clinton plan available at that point said flatly that it would allow states or local purchasing alliances to offer just one health plan of their choosing. Everyone in the area would have to use it. It might be a single HMO, for example, with a closed panel of doctors, which would mean essentially that no one in the state (or alliance) could ever see a doctor or use a hospital that was not on that list, unless the plan gave them special permission to do so. Nelson argued that it was not fair to deny Americans all choice in this matter. While people might be perfectly happy in most cases to restrict themselves to whichever doctors their plans designated, what if they occasionally wanted to pay a little more to consult a doctor who was not on the list? Nelson proposed that every health plan should offer individuals the option of such a "point-of-service" plan, a reference to the fact that patients could decide when they needed medical service whether they wanted to go to an outside doctor. After extensive discussion, the group unanimously agreed to endorse Nelson's proposal. A position paper explaining the idea was drawn up after the meeting and circulated in Washington. The White House later endorsed the idea, though the president's proposal does not require states to follow it.

That is the way Jackson Hole's influence works, slowly, through carefully explained arguments and voluminous economic and health data, month after month, year after year. No one in the group is an elected official. But quiet persuasion has convinced the governors of dozens of states and business groups in more than 150 cities, as well as the leaders of both political parties, that the Jackson Hole ideas have merit. Dr. Ellwood is constantly on the road, explaining the ideas to health providers and business groups around the country and soliciting information about local methods in hopes of advancing his own knowledge. Sometimes, in fact, it seems that he does not spend much more time in Jackson Hole than his guests do. In 1992, and again in 1993, he traveled more than 300,000 miles to discuss health-care reform. "That's an awful lot of rotaries and Chambers of Commerce," he quips. Even so, it is always difficult to be certain what he is accomplishing. "This industry is of such scale and complexity," he says, "that it is very hard to tell, sometimes, whether you've made any progress at all. It's not like being a surgeon, and you go in and they're dead, and you stick a tube down their throats and they suddenly breathe. You never really know whether or not you are breathing life into the health system."

Paul Ellwood was a young doctor running a hospital in Minnesota in the 1960s when he became convinced that American medicine was desperately in need of a cure. The hospital had been a polio unit when he joined it in the 1950s as a new graduate of the Stanford Medical School. After the polio epidemic ended, the hospital specialized in rehabilitation services as the Sister Kenny Institute. Ellwood, a pediatric neurologist, soon learned that a hospital that serves its patients too well can get into financial difficulty pretty fast. Health insurance reimbursed hospitals according to how long patients stayed in them, rather than paying for successful treatment. The financial incentives of hospital insurance were undermining the main goal of rehabilitative medicine: to make the patients self-reliant as quickly as possible. The sooner a hospital could discharge its patients and move them on to complete independence, the deeper into the red it would go. "Rehabilitation was a rather primitive field when I started," he recalls, "and so patients tended to stay in the hospital a very long time. But as we got to be much better at it, we emptied out half the beds. And we started losing money, which led me to search around for other kinds of patients to put in the hospital.

"Late one night, I was making rounds and I heard all these kids crying. I went to see what was wrong. I found out it was my fault. They were so upset to be there, and I realized they didn't have to be. I had hospitalized them for treatment of learning disorders. You see, Blue Cross would pay for their testing in the hospital, but not if they were not in the hospital. I found myself thinking that this crazy way of financing health care was making me a bad doctor, and furthermore, it was not helping my patients. I realized for the first time that nobody in this system really represents the patients."[2]

Ellwood began reading about health finance and talking to other doctors distressed by its balky and illogical rules. He studied prepaid models like the Kaiser Permanente health plan, based in his hometown of Oakland. He was beginning to spend less and less time practicing medicine and virtually all of his time analyzing it. "I became a doctor because my father is a doctor, and I never wanted to be anything else. He was a family practitioner, a very idealistic man who worked in the Oakland ghetto until he was eighty-five years old. He spent most of his life working with the poor. I practiced medicine for seventeen years. I loved being a doctor. But I gradually came to believe that some doctor had to study medicine in all of its economic and political and clinical aspects and try to figure out how to improve its performance." By 1968, as executive director of the new American Rehabilitation Foundation (ARF), the research arm of the Kenny Institute near Minneapolis, Ellwood had begun a comprehensive critique of the U.S. health-care system.

Before long, an article by Robert Levine in the journal *The Public Interest* supplied him with the nub of the idea that became his touchstone: market-based medicine, firmly guided by broad public policies. Levine argued persuasively that no large, closely regulated federal system had ever worked as well as a diverse market system. Flexibility, economic self-interest, and decentralization were always key to progress in efficiency and quality.[3] As Levine saw it, government programs targeted problems and then created myriad rules to address them. But inevitably, the rules prompted inefficient behavior. Instead of rewarding results and allowing room for common sense and imaginative improvements, they defined in numbing detail the specific actions and situations for which they would pay and thus locked the systems rigidly in place.

For Ellwood, the new Medicare and Medicaid programs illustrated the pattern perfectly. They were intended to provide medical help to the poor, the disabled, and the elderly. As a hospital administrator, though, Ellwood knew that the unwieldy programs were rapidly accelerating inflationary pressures. There were no incentives for hospitals to find ways to get people better faster or to deliver health services to patients at home or in outpatient settings because under the government rules, they would not be rewarded for doing so. Therefore, hospitals were using the federal money to build new wings, buying equipment and hiring doctors, and paying for much of it by charging the government billions of dollars for keeping people in hospitals when they did not need to be there. In just four years, the government programs had doubled in cost and were pumping up medical prices throughout the U.S. health system. Everyone was paying the price for these plans, even those covered under private insurance, since the higher prices were driving up their premiums. In Washington, D.C., meanwhile, a permanent health-reform lobby made up of nonprofit think tanks and academics was trying to persuade Congress to nationalize or thoroughly regulate every aspect of the health system. The passage of Medicare and Medicaid had given this lobby heart that the rest of the American health system could eventually be brought under close government control. Ellwood believed such an approach would only drive up prices and harm quality in medicine. It would hurt the patients.

He studied market incentives, looking for ways to encourage the major financial interests in medicine — hospitals, doctors, and insurance companies — to embrace methods voluntarily that better served the public interest. He was frustrated by the intransigence of these powerful groups, which resisted the idea of change, content to keep on making money as things stood. Adopting the terminology of the antiwar movement, he began throwing around phrases like "the rehabilitation-industrial complex" in his journal articles. Within a few years, others were talking about "the medical-industrial complex." In 1967, Ellwood took on the insurance industry in a blistering monograph that told them they were far too powerful to maintain their independence indefinitely, since they controlled such a vital service: health care. He told them they had to contribute more to public needs, perhaps by providing free medical care in rural areas and inner cities. "The chairman of Metropolitan Life invited me down for a chat," he recalls. "Then they all ignored me."

Undeterred, Ellwood soon concluded from his health system research that two ideas that had been around for a while in limited application must be combined in any workable national reform: prepaid health plans and physician group practice. Doctors working together, he felt, could offer sensible and reasonably priced care for the full range of medical needs a family might have. The idea of joining prepayment with group practice had been tried during the Great Depression. But most physicians fought this "socialized" medicine. They said it would undermine their clinical independence, that it would restrict a physician's freedom to do whatever was best for patients without consulting a boss or a budget. Besides, medicine was one of the most highly respected professions. Most doctors were not ready to become hired hands.

Even in the late 1960s, as Ellwood was studying the system, little had changed. By then, only a dozen cities had limited prepaid plans. Insurance companies remained emphatically opposed to covering broad preventive care. Hospitals were not moving with any enthusiasm toward outpatient services. Most doctors still derisively referred to prepaid plans as socialized medicine, or worse. In the winter of 1970, after a few years of looking for a receptive ear for his ideas in Washington, D.C., Ellwood got a chance to make his pitch.

President Richard Nixon was talking about a "massive health-care crisis" in America. He was struggling to formulate a national policy that could expand access to health care while curbing the rapidly growing costs.[4] On February 5, 1970, Ellwood met with senior members of the Nixon administration. He argued that to achieve the president's goals, the federal government must inject competition into the health market. He pointed out that the health system paid for treating people only when they were sick and offered virtually no incentives for providing inexpensive preventive or outpatient care. People ought to pay, he said, for health maintenance, not just episodic medical intervention. If health providers were paid the same whether the patient was sick or well, they would have strong incentives to offer the kinds of preventive care that could help keep people well. He proposed that the government switch Medicare and Medicaid coverage to prepaid plans that included outpatient treatment, with an emphasis on prevention and early diagnosis. To deliver this care, he proposed local health corporations, perhaps structured as group practices or cooperatives. He dubbed them health maintenance organizations.[5]

When the Nixon administration presented its health
maintenance organization proposal to Congress, in the form
of a new Medicare Part C that would encourage Medicare
and Medicaid beneficiaries to use HMOs, the idea immediately ran into stiff opposition from congressional leaders,
labor unions, and lobbies for the American Medical Association and the American Hospital Association. After nearly
four years of battling, Nixon signed a cumbersome and
crippled version of the HMO bill on December 29, 1973.
Shortly thereafter, HMOs lost their main proponent in
Washington when the Nixon presidency collapsed over the
Watergate scandal. The new Ford administration opposed
HMOs. Ellwood, by now president of InterStudy, the nonprofit successor to the American Rehabilitation Foundation,
recalls a sense of deep dismay as he saw the promise of
reform fading.

Once Jimmy Carter succeeded Ford, though, Ellwood
found another disciple for prepaid medicine; Carter was
looking for ways of controlling federal spending without
hurting the quality of vital services like health care. He liked
what he heard about the quality and efficiency of prepaid
plans like Kaiser's. About the same time, Alain Enthoven
approached the Carter administration with an idea for a
competitive model for national health-care reform. Ellwood
and Enthoven had met in 1973 on a ski slope at Aspen and
had soon become close collaborators and friends. Ellwood
was casual, the kind of guy who liked to commute to his
suburban Minneapolis office in a canoe from his place
across Christmas Lake. Enthoven was more reserved. But
riding up on the ski lift that day, they discovered their intense mutual interest in health reform.

Enthoven had served as a cost-control expert in Robert
McNamara's Defense Department during the Vietnam War,
focusing on how to build first-rate weapons at decent cost.
In Washington, he says, he learned the hard way that effi-

ciency and common sense have nothing to do with the way the federal government spends its money. Members of Congress were always more concerned with making sure that any new federal program created jobs or preserved benefits for the people who could vote for them. Federal spending inevitably was layered with expensive favors for those who decided how and where the government got what it needed. As he puts it, "The ideal weapons system is built in 435 congressional districts, and it's really not very important whether it works, or how much it costs."[6]

Since leaving the Pentagon, Enthoven had been thinking about how to improve U.S. medicine. As he saw it, medicine had much in common with defense spending: there was little competition, and there were few controls over the costs. He had developed some ideas on how to use market mechanisms to encourage doctors and hospitals to provide better health care more efficiently, by changing the way they were organized and paid. Like Ellwood, Enthoven believed that doctors would behave differently if they had new kinds of financial incentives that rewarded them for keeping people healthy and curbing the costs of care. If they did not earn more money every time they ordered up a test, they would not do so many unnecessary things for patients. The systems analyst became the economics half of the new partnership: Ellwood knew medicine, but Enthoven knew how markets work.

President Carter rejected Enthoven's plan, in part because he favored a more regulatory approach to reform. He was also busy coping with the larger problems then battering the economy. Once again, the vision of national reform fizzled. But the market-based approach caught the imagination of many reformers around the country. Ellwood and Enthoven now had the basic idea for what they would later call "managed competition."

Enthoven recalls their thinking: "The only forces known

to man that really reduce costs are market forces and competition. We did not advocate a pure, free-market approach to medicine, because we felt it was very important to be sure that doctors and hospitals did not just compete on price, but also provided the best possible quality to their patients. We thought it was very important to lay down some fair rules so that everyone could get affordable insurance coverage. Paul and I believed that we could get better-quality medical care in the United States at lower cost if we just had integrated, organized health systems that worked, for example, the way Kaiser does, with doctors committed to working together as a team, and learning from one another how to do a better job for patients."[7]

The two men had begun talking about these ideas with doctors, hospital administrators, insurance executives, and corporate managers responsible for employee health coverage during occasional weekends at Ellwood's vacation place in Jackson Hole, and continued the meetings in Ellwood's new home there after he moved to Wyoming. Ellwood was promoting something he called a preferred provider organization, essentially a managed-care plan run by a group of physicians and, sometimes, hospitals. It was something like the Kaiser system but could be smaller and more flexible.

The U.S. Chamber of Commerce encouraged business to try Ellwood's ideas. Companies began to sign up their employees in managed-care plans to save money.[8] Hawaii established a loosely regulated, market-based system much like the model the Jackson Hole Group was developing. Hawaiian officials had liked President Nixon's ideas for health reform and had borrowed much of their plan from the writings of Ellwood and like-minded thinkers.[9] Minnesota moved rapidly into managed care. Several former researchers from Ellwood's InterStudy institute headed HMOs in the state.[10] Other states began to experiment with the evolving Jackson Hole approach.

Today, one of the largest systems using a version of managed competition is in California, where state employees get
their medical care through health co-ops. Once a year,
everyone has the opportunity to change plans and try
something else. Enthoven notes that the system offers all of
the workers more individual choices, while controlling the
costs through cooperative purchasing. Employees of tiny
departments in remote areas have as much choice as those
in huge urban agencies. Enthoven says: "My favorite example is the Mosquito Abatement District of Antelope Valley,
California. They have two employees. Now, picture the situation as seen by those two mosquito-abaters. Once a year,
they get the brochure that describes all of the available
plans in the state and their premiums. And each of them
gets to choose a health plan. One of them can say, 'I want to
be with the Blue Shield HMO,' and the other one can say,
'Well, I want to be with HealthNet or Kaiser.' It works." Enthoven says that small businesses with only a handful of
employees could enjoy the same sort of expanded choice
and low prices if a national managed-competition system is
put in place.

Over the years, managed care has caught on more slowly
in the private sector. One reason: employers hobbled HMO
growth because of the way they set up the plans. First, most
companies allowed their workers to decide whether to keep
their familiar fee-for-service coverage or try out one of the
new HMOs. Then they gave employees no financial incentive to choose the HMO.

Employers stood to gain if workers enrolled in HMOs.
Typically, companies paid more for fee-for-service coverage,
in which employees could choose their own doctors without restriction, than for managed-care plans. Fee-for-
service doctors are paid for every service they provide, and
tend to do more for patients than managed-care physicians
usually do. The HMO premiums tend to be lower. But if the

company saved money when workers joined an HMO, the workers usually did not see the savings; the employee share of the costs was usually the same either way. Since the employees did not save any money by joining the HMO, people who might have tried the new plans decided to keep their traditional coverage.

Aside from financial considerations, most people were reluctant to join a health-care plan that could restrict a doctor's decisions on treatment. Who wanted to answer to those bean counters when something as serious as medical need was at stake? Nobody had ever heard of a doctor having to call some accountant somewhere before you could go to the hospital. It seemed downright un-American. When you were sick, you wanted to call the best doctor you knew, and get some help. But the cost-conscious health plans had introduced a third wheel into the doctor-patient relationship that set everyone's teeth on edge. They called them "gate keepers." Sometimes they were the primary care physicians or nurses in the plans who dealt with patients directly, but sometimes they were just a voice on the phone. They decided who could go through the budget "gate" to specialists, surgeons, and expensive diagnostic tests — and who could not. There was much discussion of the chilling new term. It had a strange resonance. "What are they talking about?" said one uncomfortable patient. "Pearly gates? Cattle gates?" In the cattle business, someone recalled, they had gate keepers like this, who sort out the animals for slaughter. In the lexicon of management, however, the gate keeper is the dispassionate bureaucrat who gives thumbs-up or thumbs-down on decisions regarding the allocation of resources: what to buy, which projects to nurture or drop, which budgets to trim. He keeps his eye on the big picture, and makes the pieces fit.

After years of trial and error, the quality of treatment offered in managed-care plans still varies widely. Some offer first-rate care through closely analyzed and reasonable management of treatment. California's Kaiser, Pennsylvania's U.S. Healthcare, Utah's Intermountain Health Care, and the Harvard Community Health Plan in Massachusetts are among the many institutions that have proved that excellence can be achieved in managed care. Even the Mayo Clinic, the gold standard of medicine, is now in the managed-care business. All of these plans emphasize the importance of preventive care in keeping people healthier.

Howard Godnick could not agree more with that idea. He likes to say he owes his life to the bean counters of managed care. A muscular thirty-five-year-old Brooklyn attorney who is devoted to fitness, Godnick had not consulted a doctor in years, but anyone could see that he was in great shape. After all, he ran marathons and worked out nearly every day. In the spring of 1993, though, his law firm changed health plans, signing up with a managed-care firm. As a new enrollee, Godnick took a physical. He was irritated. "I went down for the five-dollar checkup," he growls, "and they said something didn't look right." Further testing showed that all of Godnick's major heart arteries were blocked. "If it hadn't been for that physical, I would have been dead by now," he says. "There's no doubt about it. I would have gone out jogging one morning and dropped dead of a gigantic heart attack." In July of 1993, Godnick had multiple-bypass surgery at New York Hospital in Manhattan. In August, he took his family to the beach for a vacation. By September, he was back at work and also back to jogging. He plans to compete in the 1994 New York City marathon.

While Godnick is an extraordinary example of the value of the preventive care offered by HMOs, sometimes the financial arrangements in these plans encourage doctors to practice second-rate medicine. Under a practice known as "specialty capitation," for example, groups of specialists under contract to a hospital or health plan agree in advance to treat patients for a flat annual fee, regardless of the actual amount of care they deliver. Therefore, they make more profit if they do less. Unlike the broad-based prepaid plans, which can average the financial consequences of decisions on how to care for individual patients over a wide range of treatment, these groups are setting annual caps for specific kinds of services. Problems arise when their negotiated fee is too low to allow for responsible decisions, or when they simply behave in an unethical manner to save money. Some HMOs and other managed-care plans withhold up to 20 percent of their physicians' annual compensation, paying the "withhold" at the end of the year only if the doctors have stayed within tight budget targets in treating their patients. The doctors therefore have a direct financial incentive to do less for their patients.

If the physician group is large, the budget is sensible, and the management values are sound, the difference in the cost of treating individual patients may be negligible. Trouble is more likely when management is interested only in the bottom line and isn't smart enough to get there without compromising quality. Physicians working in poorly managed HMOs admit that they sometimes feel peer pressure to deny care that they feel a patient needs. Says one HMO doctor in Los Angeles: "It's scary. One very sick patient can blow the budget and chop everyone's income." Others complain that their plans budget the time they can spend with patients so closely that they fear they may be missing signs of trouble that they really should catch. When that happens, the plans destroy a key element of good medicine: listening to the patient. The doctor who has no time to listen may have no idea what is really wrong.

When seriously ill patients are referred to specialists who are not employed by the plan, conflicts often arise between the gate keeper and the outside doctor. A distraught San Francisco oncologist reported the troubles he had getting permission from a gate keeper so one of his cancer patients could come to him for the necessary follow-up visits after major surgery. He told her to come six times over a period of months. The gate keeper — a staff doctor in the patient's health plan — told him that she could only come twice. The oncologist insisted that, considering the extremely serious nature of the surgery and the importance of monitoring possible recurrences, six visits were needed. The staff doctor responded: "Two are enough." The plan's budget would not cover any more.

Ellwood and Enthoven had worried about a market-based health system that competed only on price. Unless health plans were accountable for their quality, price wars could degrade medical care. Ellwood also wanted to improve the flow of information among physicians so that they could learn from one another how to do a good job more efficiently. He wanted to know how many patients make full recoveries and are able to resume their normal activities. What really works best? Nobody was keeping track of the results. He had taken a stab at getting the insurance industry to organize such research with his 1967 monograph. In it, he had urged the insurance companies to create a prestigious industry-wide health system research center modeled on Bell Labs that would study the best ways to care for patients. As the payers of medical bills, the insurance companies would be in a position to solicit information from the doctors and hospitals. When the insurers showed no interest in his idea, Ellwood devoted his InterStudy group to such research. He has steadily convinced a number of large employers that they should keep track of quality by including patient questionnaires in their health plans.[11] But he will not be satisfied until all health providers contribute to such quality research. He may get there soon: most of the leading proposals for health-care reform, including the Clinton plan, incorporate some form of that idea.

Ellwood and Enthoven have come a long way in the twenty years since that ski-lift conversation in Aspen. Sitting in his living room last August and looking back on the early Jackson Hole gatherings, Ellwood laughed: "At first, I couldn't get anyone to come! They didn't see why they should." One by one, though, the heads of the AMA, the Mayo Clinic, and Kaiser, along with other key health and political leaders, followed the gravel road up the mountain to Ellwood's place and even donned beat-up cowboy hats from his sweat-stained collection of antiques when it was time for the barbecue. Rural health organizations and other consumer groups sent representatives. Only one key American health interest has resisted all of Ellwood's entreaties to participate in these confabs. "I've invited organized labor to almost every meeting," he says. "They've never come."

Building its influence gradually, the Jackson Hole Group has developed a formidable chess-style offense to advance its ideas, with pieces attacking Capitol Hill from every direction. Ellwood and Enthoven have built influential strongholds espousing their philosophy of market-based reform not only throughout the health system, but also in the boardrooms of corporate America, in Chambers of Commerce, think tanks, city halls, and statehouses across the country. All of these power players, at every level, will have a say in any national reform. Many of them speak Ellwood's language.

Moreover, as Congress searches for a workable compromise, nearly all of the competing proposals for health-care reform, from the Republican Senate plan led by Rhode Island's John Chafee to the White House approach, are based on the precepts of Jackson Hole. The key exception, the single-payer proposal, which would put the federal government in charge of all health care and finance it through large tax increases, seems at this point to have little chance of becoming law. Several leading congressional proponents of the single-payer approach, including California congressman Pete Stark, endorsed the White House plan when it was submitted as legislation. Growled Stark: "I kissed a frog. And it was still a frog." But before endorsing the Clinton plan, the single-payer proponents had greatly influenced its shape, winning many concessions from the White House expanding government controls over medicine. As a congressional voting bloc key to President Clinton's success, they hope to win still more concessions along the way, so that any final bill will look more to them like a prince than a frog. But they face stiff opposition on Capitol Hill. For the moment at least, the ideas of managed competition dominate the debate.

In the offices of the Jackson Hole Group in Ellwood's home, there is scant evidence of the importance of the organization in the movement for national reform. The library is well stocked, but it leans heavily to natural science (everything you might want to know about African wildlife or birds found in the Rockies, for instance), and includes only a handful of books on health policy. Over the years, Ellwood has won several prestigious awards for his research; they are tucked out of sight behind pictures of his children. Hidden on the wall behind one stack of documents is a mass-produced, machine-signed card from Bill Clinton thanking him for his "valuable contributions." Ellwood finds it amusing. Forget the trappings of influence: when it comes to health policy, he cares only about results. And if the effort to pass a national reform law should fail? "I will never give up," he says, with uncharacteristic force. "I'll just shift my attention to the states. I think they understand our ideas."

6

THE CLINTON PLAN

LATE in the summer of 1993, the *New Yorker* magazine ran a cartoon that summed up the impatience that many Americans were beginning to feel as they waited for the White House to tell them how it would fix the health-care system. On a television in a darkened living room, a newsman announces: "Finally, today, President Clinton has revealed his long-awaited health-care package." Perched in the armchair facing the television is the skeleton of a long-dead viewer.

In fact, it took the president only nine months to craft his health-care proposal. But it seemed longer. After thousands of news stories and daily White House pronouncements about the need for change and the imminent unveiling of the president's reform ideas, many Americans were tired of waiting for The Plan. The president probably understood that. And so, instead of simply sending his Health Security Act up to Capitol Hill in the normal fashion, on October 27, 1993, President Clinton and First Lady Hillary Rodham Clinton added some pizzazz to the occasion by delivering the 1,342-page document personally. Most of the members of the 103rd Congress turned out to greet them in Statuary

Hall at the Capitol, where the president made a brief speech. Pounding the lectern, he insisted that now there was no reason why the Congress could not pass a reform bill "lickety-split!" But he also appealed to the members to come forward with their own good ideas if they felt they could improve on his 240,000-word plan. Only one central idea really mattered to him, the president said: universal coverage for all Americans. He would not sign a bill unless it guaranteed every American comprehensive benefits that could never be taken away. The president stated: "That is my bottom line."

The Clinton bill finally put on paper precisely what the president wanted to do. And whatever compromises may lie ahead, as the document that may lead to national health insurance for all Americans after more than sixty years of debate, it is well worth taking a look at.

THE BASICS
Health Security

Under the plan, all Americans would be promised health-care coverage, whether they were rich or poor, employed or jobless, healthy or sick — and whether they wanted it or not. Health-care coverage would be a new right, as well as a new obligation of citizenship. Everyone would be guaranteed a standard package of comprehensive benefits and would have to contribute toward the cost of medical care. The coverage would include two broad categories of treatment: emergency care, such as hospitalization and surgery, and preventive care that could be expected to promote improved health. No one would have to worry anymore about losing insurance coverage. The benefits would be portable, meaning that Americans would keep them even if they were laid off, changed jobs, got sick, or moved to another state. No one could be denied coverage because of poor health or poverty, and no one could be dropped by an insurer. President Clinton called it "Healthcare that is always there."

The Benefits

Children receive the most sweeping protection under the Clinton plan. For the first time, all American children would be covered for physician checkups, eyeglasses, and preventive dental care, such as regular visits to a dentist and treatment of cavities. By contrast, adults would have some limited dental coverage, but primarily for emergencies.

Everyone would have greater access to other kinds of preventive medical care. These benefits would include physical examinations by doctors, for example; as things now stand, most insurance companies fully reimburse the cost of physicals only if the doctor has good reason to suspect that the patient may have a medical problem that needs to be checked. Women would be covered for occasional mammograms to check for signs of breast cancer, another examination that insurers are often reluctant to reimburse fully unless the patient has a family history of breast cancer. Women would also get regular Pap smears to check for cervical cancer. Prenatal care would be covered for expectant mothers.

Physician fees and hospitalization would be covered. So would many outpatient treatments, such as kidney dialysis, chemotherapy, radiology, biopsies, simple day surgeries, and occupational and physical therapy.

The White House proposal would ensure everyone some mental health coverage. People who already have such coverage, though, might find that the president's plan offers fewer benefits than their present plan. Under the Clinton proposal, limited outpatient treatment is stressed. If necessary, patients would be covered for up to sixty days a year of psychiatric hospitalization. Drug and alcohol rehabilitation are included but are generally limited to brief periods of outpatient therapy. Hillary Clinton calls this "a good start."

For the first time, Medicare recipients would be reimbursed for their prescriptions, after paying an annual deductible. That benefit will be very important to the elderly Americans who have difficulty paying sometimes as much as several thousand dollars a year for multiple maintenance medications.

Women would be covered for prescription birth control devices as well as abortions. In vitro fertilization would not be covered.

Disabled Americans would be reimbursed for some prosthetic devices, such as leg braces and wheelchairs. Those who suffer from severe chronic illnesses would be covered for some home health services, such as receiving medications or nutrients through intravenous tubes, if the patient would otherwise have to go to the hospital for the treatment. Most insurance policies do not currently include those services. People with terminal illnesses such as AIDS and cancer would be covered for some hospice care; that would be a great help to dying people who can no longer stay in the hospital and need some care in their final days.

Among the other medical items that would not be covered are hearing aids and eyeglasses for adults. Nor would national health insurance reimburse people for orthodontic dental care or private duty nurses or most cosmetic surgery.

The New Health-Care System

To provide health care, the Clinton proposal borrows from the Jackson Hole plan. Independent insurance agents would be obsolete, for the most part, because almost everyone would be required to join purchasing cooperatives that would negotiate health coverage for them and handle the payments. President Clinton calls these co-ops "alliances." Individuals and companies would pay their insurance premiums to these alliances, which would then pay the doctors, HMOs, and other health providers. Only employers with 5,000 or more workers could choose to set up their own, separate health alliances for their employees. By collecting people into such large groups, the White House aims to achieve the Jackson Hole goal of giving people greater bargaining power with physicians and other providers so that they can obtain affordable coverage. But the Clinton plan makes the middleman — or alliance — far more powerful and regulatory than the authors of managed competition envisioned. Under the White House proposal, these alliances would tend to be very large. Many of them would operate as state agencies; some would enjoy a monopoly on medical demand within the state because they would represent all potential patients.

In order to win the right to serve the people in these alliances, doctors, hospitals, and other health professionals would band together in large groups, or health-care plans, and compete for the alliance business. An alliance would shop around among these health-care plans comparing quality, services, price, and consumer satisfaction, then choose one or more to serve its members. Each person in the alliance would then choose a plan from that list. In most cases, people would be able to choose among a low-cost HMO type of plan, a higher-cost plan that allowed them more choice of physicians and hospitals, or a midpriced plan with moderate restrictions on individual choice. Some alliances, however, would offer only one plan for an entire state or region, and could decide which physicians and hospitals were eligible to serve all of their patients. In these cases, such alliances essentially would run health services in their regions, instead of simply negotiating with different health plans as a middleman for the consumers.

The secretary of Health and Human Services would decide what kinds of information the health plans must report to alliances.

Medicare and Medicaid would slowly be merged into the alliance system. Those who are already in the Medicare system when the new plan takes effect could choose to continue getting their benefits from the Medicare program. Those arriving at Medicare age after that would receive their care through the alliances.

Everyone Must Pay

Since some people, especially the young, have no interest in obtaining health insurance, the only way to achieve universal health coverage is to force everybody to take it. President Clinton would require everyone to buy health insurance. For the first time, companies would be told which benefits to offer and forced to pay most of the cost of health care for their full-time employees. They would also be required to provide the same benefits to part-time workers. Until now, companies have offered such benefits voluntarily, usually only to permanent full-timers, and have cut benefits at will. Under the Clinton plan, employers would pick up 80 percent of the cost of health services for full-timers. Those employees would pay the remaining 20 percent, plus the cost of deductibles and moderate cash payments for doctor appointments, prescriptions, and other health services.

To ease the significant new costs to employers, the government would subsidize some of them. No company participating in an alliance, for instance, would pay more than 7.9 percent of payroll costs for employee health care; if prices rose faster than salaries (as they have for half a century or more), the taxpayers would make up the difference.

Taxpayers would also help out with the new bur
ering the part-timers. The government would pick
centage of the cost, depending on how many ho
employee worked; the employer would pay the rest.
payers would also subsidize insurance for people whose
comes fall below 150 percent of the poverty line and for
employee coverage at the smallest firms.

Self-employed Americans would be required to buy coverage. They could deduct the full cost of the insurance from
their taxes. People who don't work would also have to buy
coverage unless they qualified for government health coverage. It is not clear, though, how the government can
make many of the unemployed buy insurance.

Under a system called "community rating," everyone in a
health plan would pay the same insurance premiums, regardless of their medical condition. In effect, younger and
healthier people, who seldom see a doctor, would subsidize
the heavier usage of medical services by sicker, disabled, or
older people. This also means that no one would have to
fear a sudden hike in insurance premiums if he or she or a
family member became seriously ill.

Government Price Controls

In its broad outlines, the Clinton proposal may have been
drawn loosely from the Jackson Hole model of managed
competition, but the White House made fundamental
changes, relying on regulation more than market forces.
Most important, the Clinton proposal would dramatically
expand government regulatory power over medicine and
would establish a complex series of new price controls.

Under the plan, a new National Health Board, part of the
executive branch of government, would decide how much
to spend on health care each year. The Board would then
tell each alliance around the country how much it should

plan to spend taking care of its people. If medical needs and spending looked as if they were going to exceed the budget, the alliance would have the power to delay payments to doctors and other health professionals or to make automatic cuts in what they are paid. The alliance could set doctors' fees; in many cases it would be illegal for patients to pay them more than the official price.

The plan would tightly control increases in other medical prices as well, through national regulations on health costs. In the first year the national system is in effect, which the president assumes will be 1997, health insurance premiums would only be allowed to rise by the same amount as the U.S. cost of living (the consumer price index, or CPI) plus 1.5 percent. In other words, if U.S. inflation is 4 percent in 1997, health premiums could rise by no more than 5.5 percent. The second year, premiums could rise as much as the consumer price index plus 1 percent. If national inflation were 4 percent, health premiums could rise by 5 percent. By the fourth year (2000 A.D.), premiums would only be allowed to rise as much as the CPI, thus locking health-care spending into pace with basic national inflation. Considering that health inflation has been running at several times the level of U.S. inflation, this rapid racheting down would force sharp adjustments in how much time doctors spent with patients and in decisions on when people could get tests, medications, and surgery. It would be up to the doctors and nurses to figure out how to take care of everyone within the tight new budgets, even if they had to restrict services to patients or work for free to make ends meet.

Administration and Regulation

The president would appoint members of the National Health Board. The alliances would be run by political appointees chosen by the governors. The federal government would wield other broad new powers in health care. The National Health Board would say which benefits Americans would get, deciding for instance whether everyone had the right to a new treatment for cancer or some other disease. The secretary of Health and Human Services would approve the prices for new drugs and would have extensive regulatory power over the medical professions. The secretary would control how many students could choose a particular medical specialty, such as cardiology or ophthalmology, and could also set racial quotas for medical students allowed to study each physician specialty.

Family Doctors

After covering the uninsured and controlling costs, the third most important goal of health-care reform is expanding access to family doctors. The Clinton plan would offer doctors tax incentives to practice in what are called "underserved areas," primarily places in the inner cities and in rural America that do not have enough physicians. Most health experts agree that the United States needs substantially more family physicians. Only 30 percent of U.S. doctors currently practice what is commonly called primary care — that is, broad family practice, caring for everyone from infants to the elderly — though that proportion rises to nearly 45 percent when gynecologists, obstetricians, pediatricians, and general internists are counted as family doctors.[1] Under the Clinton bill, medical schools would be required to produce a minimum of 55 percent of their graduates in the basic areas of family practice, general internal medicine, general pediatrics, obstetrics, and gynecology.

To enhance access to family doctors, the administration is also counting on a little-known provision of the North American Free Trade Agreement. Under NAFTA, visa restrictions will be eased for Mexican doctors wishing to practice in the United States.

Malpractice Reform and Other Litigation

The Clinton plan takes only the most tentative steps to reform the legal system or to discourage lawsuits against doctors or other health service providers. In fact, when all aspects of the proposal are considered, it seems to expand the potential for medical litigation. Most important: the plan makes health care a broad new right. That right has yet to be defined clearly (when does a doctor have a right to say no?), which means that lawyers will try to define the right by suing doctors and health plans for infringing upon it in various ways. Under the Clinton plan, individuals will be free to sue everyone in the health-care system, right up to the secretary of Health and Human Services, if they feel that they have not been given benefits or services to which they are entitled. Under the plan, personal injury lawyers would be forbidden to charge more than 33⅓ percent of the final settlement amount in a malpractice case — but that is the amount that personal injury lawyers usually claim now.

Paperwork

The administration would seek to reduce the $100 billion or so in the health-care system's annual administrative costs by simplifying the paperwork. The plan requires that all insurers use the same claims forms, which should make it easier for doctors and others to handle the bills. At the same time, of course, the extensive new regulatory powers of the federal health agencies and the alliances are bound to generate many new kinds of paperwork.

How to Pay for It

How much will all of this cost? Estimates from respected sources vary. The White House says its plan would add about $400 billion to federal spending during the first five years, or $80 billion per year. But experts outside the administration, including members of Congress, think the new costs may be at least twice as high. Senator Daniel Patrick Moynihan of New York, the chairman of the Senate Finance Committee, has called the White House estimates "fantasy." Congressman Jim Cooper, a Tennessee Democrat, says, "I don't know anybody who thinks the costs will be that low." Cooper, who has introduced his own reform legislation, says the Clinton plan will add $1 trillion to federal spending over five years ($200 billion per year).[2]

Whatever its cost, the administration proposes to pay for the new plan by squeezing savings out of the health-care system, mainly by cutting $238 billion from Medicaid and Medicare during the first five years and by curbing waste, fraud, and what it believes are excess profits. Some of these federal savings are achieved by making the local alliances pay for things like treatment of the poor and the chronically ill that the federal government now covers.[3] These savings are, in effect, new local taxes. By shifting many Medicaid patients into local alliances, for instance, the federal government expects to save about $80 billion over five years; that $80 billion, of course, would be added to the health insurance costs of the people in the communities where those poor people live. Similarly, the administration estimates that Medicare can save $28 billion over five years by requiring Medicare beneficiaries who have jobs, or whose spouses work, to get their insurance from the employers instead of from the government. Those five million Americans would be added to the corporate health burden.[4] In addition, Medicare premiums would rise sharply for anyone with more than $90,000 in taxable income per year ($115,000 in the case of joint returns). The increases would vary according to the level of income.[5]

The Clinton plan will also levy other new taxes. Consumers will pay a new 75-cent health tax on each pack of cigarettes. Big companies will be expected to pay 7.9 percent of payroll covering their own workers; in addition, those that choose to provide employee coverage by setting up their own health-care plans will also pay a 1 percent payroll tax to subsidize the people in the local alliance. Employees would be taxed for any health benefits offered by their companies that exceed the value of the basic federal benefit package; if a company offers its workers coverage for regular dental checkups, for instance, which are not included in the Clinton plan, the workers will be taxed. There would be new taxes on sub-chapter S corporations and limited partnerships.

The administration is also considering a tax on hospitals, though it was not in the proposal submitted to Congress. Administration officials say it is part of a backup financing plan and may be added to the bill if the White House proposal falls short. Other parts of the Clinton financing are based on assumptions, perhaps unrealistically optimistic, about how the plan would affect the U.S. economy. The administration calculates, for instance, that it will collect $51 billion in new taxes because companies will be more profitable (and pay more taxes). Their reasoning: the health plan should make medicine more efficient and eventually reduce the cost to companies of employee health benefits. *The bottom line:* The plan would offer near-universal coverage, comprehensive benefits, and insurance reform but would introduce heavy regulation, higher taxes, and corporate costs; most likely, it would increase inefficiency in health care by removing some strong existing incentives to produce savings and by closely defining how providers must behave.

THE RIVAL PROPOSALS

President Clinton has created the momentum for substantial health-care reform. He has convinced the American people that it can be done, and he is determined to sign a national reform bill in 1994. But which bill? Several other legislative proposals for reform are competing with the president's plan in the Congress, and each of them has substantial support. They range from one that would place the government in charge of all health care to several that would mostly limit themselves to tinkering with ways to help people buy health insurance. Many members of Congress say that the White House proposal must undergo extensive revision before an acceptable bill can be produced. They and their advisers believe that one of the other leading proposals may provide the blueprint for the amended reform bill that can win majority support.

Here are the highlights of the alternatives:

The Single-Payer Plan

The American Health Security Act, supported by about ninety members of Congress, represents the most radical and, in some ways, the simplest suggestion for reform. This is nationalized medicine. Under the single-payer model, the government would pay for all health services (hence the name single payer), and would levy taxes to pay for them. New payroll taxes of at least 7.9 percent would be added, for instance, as well as higher corporate and personal income taxes. Everyone would be entitled to the same benefits. The federal government would regulate all aspects of medicine, from setting physician fees to deciding which operations, drugs, or diagnostic machines would be available for patient care. As proof that such a system would work, supporters point to Canada, which has had a single-payer medical system for about twenty years. They don't mention Canada's heavy tax burden, though, or its deepening problems in paying for its medical system.

Proponents of an American single-payer system emphasize several advantages. It guarantees universal coverage, for one thing. Because companies would no longer be the source of health coverage for workers, a single-payer plan would eliminate people's worries about losing insurance when they lose their jobs, or when they move from a large company to a small firm. Such a system would also eliminate much of the paperwork that is generated when many insurance companies with different rules use a dizzying array of forms. Under the single-payer plan, there would be one set of rules for everyone, and the insurance companies would be abolished. Supporters also argue that by closely regulating the prices charged by doctors and other providers, the plan would save money.

While the approach sounds simple enough, critics say it ignores at least two vital considerations: significantly higher taxes and lower medical quality. Nationalizing American medicine would require a vast and costly new state and federal bureaucracy and would produce a huge new tax burden that would depress economic growth. In addition, since doctors and hospitals would operate under absolute budgets, they would have to deny many services to patients as too expensive. For the same reason, new treatments might be sidelined for budget reasons, as they sometimes are in single-payer systems like Canada's. Moreover, innovation would be crippled: stripped of any financial incentives to compete or to develop breakthrough technologies and procedures, medicine would decline in quality. Investors would place their capital elsewhere, where it could make money. And in a system where the government tells providers exactly how much it intends to spend, no one has an incentive to do a better job for less.

Nevertheless, the single-payer plan has great appeal, because it sounds safe. Hoping to defuse its popularity and to win support from its proponents, President Clinton added several key characteristics of the single-payer approach to his own proposal. Examples include his price controls and premium limits, as well as the huge and bureaucratic new alliances that would control health care. Most important, though, is a provision of the Clinton plan that permits any state to declare itself a single-payer state and offer only one, state-controlled medical plan. When the president's plan was introduced as legislation, it was endorsed by several leading supporters of the single-payer approach. As much as anything, that was a courtesy; they will continue to press forward with their own proposal.

The bottom line: Universal coverage, comprehensive benefits, elimination of the insurance industry, high taxes, lower quality, and less medical care.

The Cooper Plan

Congressman Jim Cooper, a Tennessee Democrat, first introduced his Managed Competition Act during election year 1992, nearly a year before President Clinton submitted his own plan to Congress. Cooper's plan resembles the president's proposal in many ways, but it is simpler, more economical, and less regulatory. Cooper calls it "Clinton Lite."

Cooper's managed-competition proposal would guarantee access to health coverage for Americans but would not require everyone to buy it. Most people would join local Jackson Hole–style health cooperatives and would choose from a list of competing health plans. Unlike the Clinton alliances, Cooper's would have no broad regulatory powers but would simply operate as insurance buyers, bargaining for better quality and prices on behalf of local residents. Companies with a hundred or more employees would be allowed to set up their own independent health alliances if they preferred to do so. Everyone would be offered comprehensive health benefits, and no one could be denied insurance. The key difference between the Clinton and Cooper plans is that Clinton requires everyone to buy insurance, while Cooper does not. Clinton also requires companies to pay most of the cost of benefits. Cooper requires companies to offer benefits, but leaves it up to them to decide, as they now do, how much of the cost to bear.

Like Dr. Paul Ellwood and Professor Alain Enthoven, who favor his approach, Cooper believes that managed competition is the best way to encourage better health care at lower prices. He rejects the price controls and premium caps in the Clinton plan, arguing that they would only hurt quality, increase inefficiency (and therefore costs), and discourage competition. He also believes that while the government should make it possible for everyone to afford decent health insurance, it is not the role of government to force them to buy it. Cooper says that would make health care a full-blown entitlement, leading to more medical inflation and inefficiency, and destroying jobs as smaller companies struggled to pay the bills. Instead, Cooper focuses on making it easier for individuals to afford insurance, through community rating and increased competition among providers for the right to serve the small local alliances. He argues that health reform should attack the most pressing problem first — covering those Americans who cannot afford insurance. As he puts it, "I think that our bill is about as ambitious as we can afford to be right now." Cooper notes that Clinton's plan is more than four times as long as his. Instead of just fixing the problems, he says, Clinton would impose complex new rules on every part of medicine.

The price tag? In 1992, the Congressional Budget Office, the economic analysis arm of Congress, estimated the cost of implementing Cooper's system at $25 billion a year. But Cooper thinks that is a bit low. He says his plan may cost closer to $40 billion a year, though that is still only a small fraction of the cost of the White House plan.[6] The plan seems to be the main rival to President Clinton's, since Cooper has attracted broad bipartisan support in both houses of Congress.

The bottom line: Universal access to coverage, dramatically less regulation than in the Clinton plan, comprehensive benefits, affordable insurance, lower health costs, an emphasis on individual responsibility and choice, and spirited competition among providers.

The Chafee Plan

Introduced by Rhode Island's John Chafee, the Senate Republican Health Care Task Force plan, which is cosponsored by minority leader Robert Dole and about twenty other Republican senators, proposes a different way to achieve universal coverage. Like the Clinton and Cooper proposals, the Chafee plan is based on managed competition and offers everyone a comprehensive package of health benefits. But no American would be forced to participate in its local alliances. Individuals and companies with a hundred or fewer employees would be welcome to take advantage of the bargaining power represented by the alliances. Requirements for everyone to obtain some kind of insurance coverage would be phased in over several years. The federal government would subsidize insurance for the poor.

Savings on health costs would come from stepping up pressure on health providers to compete for the right to serve patients in the alliances. But those savings would probably not be nearly as great as those that could be achieved under the Cooper plan, since many companies and individuals would probably decline to participate in the cost-conscious voluntary alliances.

The government would finance the costs of the plan, in part, by eliminating the dollar-for-dollar tax deduction that large employers now take for providing employee health care; the write-off is a major incentive to provide such benefits. This is a question of fairness. Under existing tax law, small firms do not enjoy the 100 percent write-off when they provide benefits to their workers. Moreover, workers at smaller companies, many of whom do not get employee benefits, support the generous coverage of the employees of big companies through their taxes. In another move toward fairness, Chafee would also tax workers for the value of any employee benefits over and above those in the package guaranteed to all Americans. The reasoning: the extra benefits are like extra income, which should be taxed.

The bottom line: Phased-in universal coverage, insurance reform, greater tax fairness, a reliance on individual responsibility and choice, moderate health-care savings, and some increased competition among health providers.

The House Republican Plan

Sponsored by House minority leader Bob Michel, this proposal requires employers to set up health plans but does not require them to pay for the coverage. Employees can decide whether to get their health benefits through the company plan, in which case they might have to pay the full cost. Workers could establish medical savings accounts, something like IRAs, to pay for their health insurance. No basic benefits package would be defined. Insurance companies would be required to offer reasonably priced coverage to small business. Low-income Americans would receive federal subsidies to help pay for their health insurance.

To help pay for the plan, Medicare premiums would be raised for wealthy Americans.

The bottom line: Insurance reform and greater fairness, a reliance on individual choice and responsibility, but no universal coverage and not much more competition among providers.

All of these plans will contend for dominance in the health-care reform battle that unfolds in 1994. Most heartening, all of them seek to ensure that all Americans can get health coverage. That would help to answer the most pressing need driving the movement for health reform: covering the millions of Americans who cannot afford health insurance. But the sticking points where these plans clash are of major significance. Perhaps most important, President Clinton insists that everyone must buy insurance, and employers must pay most of the cost of medical care; Jim Cooper and Bob Michel, and their groups of supporters on both sides of the aisle in the House and the Senate, strongly disagree with these Draconian requirements. Pete Stark and the other proponents of a single-payer plan want the government to pay for medicine through taxes.

In the end, it is possible that no agreement will be reached. That would fly in the face of the grassroots demand for reform. Politicians fear that voters would probably respond by exacting a high price at the polls.

More likely, the law that is passed, whether in 1994 or

later, will be a combination of the most strongly supported ideas now circulating on Capitol Hill. Many members of Congress think such a compromise might look a lot like Clinton Lite, with a few more ingredients. Will it work? A lot of Americans are beginning to worry that Congress will patch together a complex reform that may satisfy all the key political factions — but one that may also harm medical quality and cut off individual choice.

7

THOSE ENDLESS COSTS

AS the United States considers how to improve the American way of health, it faces two enormous and conflicting challenges. First, the country must find a way to contain the rapid growth of medical costs in order to free the economy from this crippling burden. But at the same time, in aiming for universal coverage, it must expand access to health care, which will drive up demand and therefore overall costs. In order to accomplish both goals, enormous discipline must be introduced into the medical system, and careful thought must be given to the way that access is expanded. Regardless of its precise form, any legislation that guarantees comprehensive health coverage to everyone will constitute the largest entitlement in American history, one that will inflate demand by elevating health care to the level of a legal right and further by guaranteeing payment of medical bills. The new system must be efficient and must have some way of ensuring value in its medical services. In shaping reform, moreover, it is important to understand not only what is pushing up costs now, but also the forces that will continue to drive up health spending for decades to come.

It is not enough to tinker with the present system to pare spending, eliminating much of the billions of dollars in annual paperwork, for example, or making individual Americans pay a greater share of the costs, necessary though both measures are. Nor is it enough to crack down on billions of dollars worth of fraud and waste in the system, though that, too, is crucial. Even if price controls worked, in fact, the runaway costs could not be contained.

It is not only the prices that are killing us. It is the rapidly growing demand for health services. And we are about to expand that demand dramatically. The danger is that a poorly designed reform plan could do enormous damage to medical quality as well as to the country's ability to sustain the availability of health services. The only way to get the costs under control is to address the underlying dynamics of American medical demand. If the uniquely American health plan promised by our leaders is to succeed, it must address uniquely American problems.

For one thing, unlike Canada, Germany, and Japan, where health spending is somewhat more moderate, the United States spends billions every year on the medical consequences of its disproportionate social ills. There is a reason, for example, why UCLA medical center and some other urban hospitals have become expert in the treatment of spinal injuries inflicted by automatic weapons: they are coping with the tragedies flowing from the bloody wars of youth gangs that are unmatched anywhere else in the industrialized world. No place in America is immune from the plague of violence anymore.

Billions of dollars in health costs are incurred when doctors and nurses treat the problems arising from poverty, homelessness, crime, violence, drug abuse, alcoholism, teen pregnancy, child neglect and abuse, and other problems largely caused by distintegrating family and community values. In 1990 alone, drug and alcohol abuse cost the

United States $166 billion, including medical treatment and other costs. Every year, alcohol and drugs lead to about 100,000 premature deaths.[1]

Heavy drinking and drug addiction lead to violence: an estimated two-thirds of all homicides and serious assaults.[2] They lead to accidents, as well as suicide, chronic liver disease, heart attack, and stroke. They also cause birth defects. One out of every five Medicaid dollars spent on hospitalization goes to treat people for conditions caused by substance abuse. Drug abuse explains more than half of all of the tragic pediatric AIDS cases.[3] Medicaid spends about $2 billion looking after the more than 150,000 babies born each year who are severely impaired by crack poisoning. Treating each baby for the first five years of his or her life costs about $63,000.[4] On average, the babies of substance-abusing mothers spend three times as long in the hospital as other babies. When children under fifteen abuse substances, they are hospitalized three to four times longer than others, regardless of the nature of their illness. Substance abuse complicates the treatment of many diseases, more than doubling the average hospital stays of patients treated for pneumonia, burns, and septicemia. Two-thirds of all strokes suffered by young Americans are related to cocaine abuse or heavy smoking.[5]

Every year, nearly one million teenagers become pregnant;[6] their babies are often premature, underweight, and sick and are far more likely to live in poverty. Every year, about the same number of teenagers drop of out of school at a time when that decision is likely to mean a life of deprivation, substandard nutrition, preventable death from heart disease and other illnesses, as well as a greater vulnerability to violent crime. If we are to ensure that full access to health services is available and affordable for all, these American social problems must be addressed.

*   *   *

More important, while the United States undertakes reform
of its health system, it must plan ahead for the epochal
change in the nature of medicine and medical need that is
creating massive new inflationary pressure. During this
century, life expectancy has jumped from forty-seven to
seventy-five years. But as the population ages, it is growing
sicker. Remember "natural causes"? Now they're treatable
conditions. The cruel irony is that because medicine has
done so much to conquer infectious disease and to repair
injuries, Americans now spend more years disabled at the
end of life. Chronic disease is becoming the central challenge of medicine. Already, the fastest-growing group in the
United States is people aged eighty years and older. Chronic
disease has multiple economic effects, not only increasing
direct medical costs, but also generating custodial costs,
since someone must care for many of these patients once
they are disabled. One in four Americans now suffer from
chronic diseases like Alzheimer's, severe asthma, osteoporosis, crippling arthritis, and congestive heart failure or
are family members responsible for the care of such patients.[7] That's just the beginning. Starting in just fifteen
years, the more than 70 million Baby Boomers will begin to
retire. As the beneficiaries of superior postwar medicine and
economic prosperity, they are expected to live longer than
their parents. That means that they will spend more years
seriously ill but in no immediate danger of dying. Medicare
and Medicaid spending are both closely tied to the problems
of aging; Medicaid pays for half of all nursing-home costs.
Within five years, the costs of these entitlements will be
greater than Social Security, accounting for nearly a third of
mandatory federal spending.

Over the next thirty years, the health system will face an
epidemic of chronic illness that could make the present national bill look like small change. Instead of focusing on attacking catastrophic illness and injury, doctors and nurses

will increasingly help patients cope with conditions that cannot be cured, that require continued treatment, and that may leave the individual somewhat debilitated, if not dependent. As medicine continues to get better at extending life, health costs will multiply. In 1987, for example, the United States spent $130 billion treating heart disease, stroke, and cancer, all of them diseases that strike heavily at advanced ages. Those costs are growing steadily. Between 1986 and 1991, the demand for echocardiograms and angioplasty (a method of clearing blockages from coronary arteries) grew by about 25 percent annually for elderly patients. In the coming years, tens of millions more will need repeated surgery, full-time custodial care, rehabilitation, physical therapy, private nursing, wheelchairs, walkers, and multiple medications. The Mayo Clinic has estimated that at least $1 billion more will be needed every year just for the additional hip replacements.

Providing coverage for the uninsured will extend their lives and healthy years, will expand their horizons, and should make them more productive, all good and valuable things. By doing so, the medical coverage will enable these Americans to live richer lives and to contribute more to the society and to economic growth. But it will also deliver millions more Americans to the long years of chronic disease and costly treatment. Though President Clinton and other political leaders are fond of defending the value of universal preventive care by claiming that it saves on overall health costs in the long run, there is no evidence to support that statement. Quite the contrary, preventive care helps to short-circuit the simpler illnesses, thankfully postponing up to 70 percent of premature deaths. But that paves the way for the more expensive illnesses later on. Dramatically fewer people die today from early heart attacks and strokes than twenty years ago, in part because so many have quit smoking and indulging in high-fat diets and because more people understand the importance of exercising and of treating conditions like high blood pressure and diabetes. There have also been impressive reductions in early deaths due to cirrhosis as Americans have reduced their consumption of hard liquor. Instead of dying sudden or early deaths, these Americans live long enough to suffer the lingering illnesses that require hundreds of thousands of dollars' worth of additional care. To take just one example, the cost of treating age-related dementia is now $100 billion a year, or one-tenth of total health spending, and it is growing.

There is no question that the responsibility of caring for the huge elderly population is going to get much harder for younger citizens to bear. Already, they resent the price they are paying in higher taxes, lower salaries, and diminished economic opportunity. If they seem unhappy to hear that the president's plan will hit their insurance costs hardest, it is because that is only the latest bill they have been handed for the support of older people. And this one's for medical care, something they hardly ever use. They look to the future, and they see social burdens and somebody's hand in their wallet. To many young Americans, the entitled elderly and the Baby Boom headed that way are beginning to seem like the monster that King Minos kept in his labyrinth, feeding it seven maidens and seven youths per year. From what they have heard about health reform, the monster's appetite is growing. They are the workers who must earn the money to keep it fed. The danger is that before long, elderly patients may be denied the care they need as the burden becomes too great for American workers to bear.

Finding more efficient ways of delivering treatment for conditions like Alzheimer's, Parkinson's disease, diabetes, arthritis, congestive heart failure, and other chronic illnesses will be key to keeping up with the rapidly growing costs. Providing government funds to put the elderly in nursing homes, for example, at present costs of up to

$50,000 per year, is not a good answer. Inevitably, families are going to have to take more responsibility for the care of their elderly, and health insurers are going to have to encourage the development of better technology and modes of home care.

Medical research will be critical to meeting this challenge. New drugs, for example, can be remarkably cost-effective for these conditions. In the summer of 1993, Parke-Davis introduced Cognex, the first pill for Alzheimer's. While Cognex does not cure the disease, it does arrest its progress for a few years in many patients. Such a pill means that patients do not lose their cognitive abilities and independence as soon, do not have to turn to custodial care. Strictly in terms of cost-effectiveness, taking Cognex will cost each patient a few hundred dollars a year, but it can save upward of $40,000 per year. Preliminary research at Duke University indicates a possible genetic explanation for much Alzheimer's disease; if the Duke researchers are right, they believe that a new drug may be devised to prevent the disease in 60 percent of cases. Unfortunately, though, there is no reliable way of predicting when scientists will find cures or other effective treatments for the chronic diseases that will disable tens of millions of Americans in the coming decades.

Meanwhile, unless reform can make health care far more efficient and accountable, the system will be in danger of slowly breaking down for lack of adequate financial support. In order to address the powerful underlying forces that will continue to fuel medical inflation, we must not only improve the present system, but must also ask what kind of system can best address the changing needs of our citizens. Other industrialized nations, including Japan and European countries, are facing the same problems of caring for a graying population. But they are coping in ways that Americans have not yet been willing to accept.

Where doctors in other countries gently inform families that there is nothing more they can do for a patient, American doctors impose massive intervention, literally unable to give up. Americans no longer accept death as a natural part of life. Patients and families are so accustomed to the extraordinary means by which doctors can defeat many life-threatening conditions that they often view death as a failure of medicine. Americans must begin to confront profound questions about the allocation of health resources and the limits of medicine. The key to doing it responsibly lies in an understanding of the mechanisms that are currently driving up costs.

At present, medical costs are propelled mainly by three powerful engines: innovation, consumer demand, and third-party reimbursement. These three factors can be described as the content of medical care, the compulsion to seek it, and the responsibility for payment. The three sources of medical inflation are closely intertwined. While physician incomes account for a bit more than 20 percent of health costs (about $200 billion), doctors control decisions for treatment that makes up 80 percent ($800 billion) of the bill. Doctors are influenced to a growing extent, as well, by consumer demand as Americans have come to believe that they have a right to everything that medicine offers. Once health care becomes a protected right, that consumer pressure on doctors will grow.

Innovation and technology helped to create that sense of the right to medical care. By its nature, medical innovation relentlessly expands the menu of available health services, even as it extends the reach of the healing art. Federal economists have estimated that new procedures add at least $12 billion every year to health costs.

Americans have enormous confidence in their doctors. Half a century ago, hospital architecture borrowed heavily from church design. The entrances to many of the great teaching hospitals built during that era are huge, vaulted cathedral archways. Just inside is a chapel. Back then, everyone had more reverence for doctors, when healing was still largely wrapped in hope and the mysteries of miracles. One entered a church to pray for help, and if it did not come, that was God's will. One entered a hospital with much the same feeling, hoping for a cure, but not assuming that it would materialize. As medicine has become more technological, though, and has extended its reach, we have come almost to assume the availability of cure. Just pick out the right pill. For Americans, confidence in science is often more powerful than religious faith. No longer the high priests of healing, physicians are now seen more as the NASA repair team, trying to save that satellite tumbling in orbit.

And no wonder: advances in medicine constantly redefine the sense of what is possible, pushing into unbelievable realms. At Columbia Presbyterian in New York City, a small British girl whose insides are all wrong gets seven transplanted organs in an unprecedented medical tour de force. During the year that she lives, she reaffirms everyone's belief that doctors can do whatever it takes to preserve one precious life. If they can do that, they must be able to do just about anything. Arlen Specter, one of the Senate's toughest debaters, has a brain tumor removed and shows up wisecracking on the Senate floor a few weeks later.

Physicians are now viewed by many people, and not only those stunned by desperate illness, as the technicians who control the keys to medicine's amazing toolbox. Doctors say that whenever newspapers report new medical breakthroughs, patients suffering from those conditions simply show up unannounced at hospitals, sometimes on stretchers or in wheelchairs.[8] Our faith in medicine masks our terror of disease and death. And the thing is, faith often works. Patients near death suddenly recover, against all odds. It isn't always medicine that brought them back. But miracles are too random and unreliable. We want to believe that medicine can stop tragedy in its tracks, and that, as much as any other reason, is why we now believe that health care is a right.

To the man who will die without a heart transplant, a heart transplant is very basic health care. To the woman who yearns for a child, infertility treatment may be what she defines as medicine to which she darn well has a right. The fifty-five-year-old demands a new and expensive form of knee surgery — not so that he can walk, but so that he can play singles.

Conditions that once were viewed as tragic or as unfortunate personal problems become insurable medical needs and produce surges in treatment. Americans have learned, for example, that drug addiction and many psychiatric problems are treatable. As a result, mental health spending is a fast-growing part of the health bill, accounting for 10 percent of the total, and mental health professionals call for "parity" in health reform, demanding universal coverage for the full range of services they provide. During the last ten years, new technology has helped surgeons make great strides in coronary bypass surgery. Surgeons are now able to take hours more to complete the operation, fixing a greater variety of problems, without damaging the heart. Understandably, a new army of patients with complex heart disease, many of them in their seventies and eighties, are demanding the operation. When all of these services are reimbursed by an insurance company, they drive up premium costs. One way or another, we all pay the bill. According to Kirk Johnson, general counsel for the American Medical Association: "The American consumer demand for health care will grow as long as people in this country want to live forever and want to do everything they can right up until the second of death. And who wants to take that away from them? How are you going to take that away? So the overall costs will increase."[9]

Medicine's costs are also irresistibly driven upward by an unusual productivity problem. For all of its impressive technology, medicine is not much more efficient than it was when doctors carried little black bags and made house calls. Economists call the problem "Baumol's disease," after the economist William J. Baumol of New York University, who first identified it in the 1960s, when medical costs were insignificant compared to today's levels.

What Professor Baumol described was a problem peculiar to so-called handicraft occupations like teaching, the performing arts, and medicine, which require a high level of personal input. He called this "the cost disease of the personal services." Unlike other industries, such as manufacturing and construction, medicine does not significantly improve its productivity when new technology is introduced. In factories, machines replace human labor and make the remaining workers more efficient. But in medicine, the modern industrial revolution that has introduced countless new treatments and services has also required innumerable new technicians and support personnel. A doctor can now obtain crystal-clear pictures of a patient's brain or spinal cord or joints with a $2 million MRI machine, but not without an MRI technician or two to run it and still other specialists to help interpret the results. The same principle holds for the $5 million PET scanner and numerous other lifesaving technologies. Many more lives are saved, but the investment in technology does not reduce the number of medical professionals necessary. The patient must be examined carefully before the precise nature of the complaint can be pinned down. New diagnostic techniques may only expand the number of steps necessary to identify the problem. Medical quality seems inextricably linked to the amount of time expended. If a doctor spends three minutes instead of fifteen on a patient visit, the patient is not getting his money's worth of that physician's attention and skills of observation. There are only so many patients a doctor can see in a day without committing medical consumer fraud.

Coronary bypass surgery and heart valve replacements have a severe case of Baumol's disease. In order to operate on the living heart, the surgeon needs the heart-lung machine, which temporarily takes over the functions of those two vital organs. Without it, the surgery would not be possible. This complex piece of machinery is operated by a perfusionist, usually a nurse with advanced technical training. Meanwhile, the patient is also kept alive and stable via a huge battery of equipment operated by the anesthesiologist, who monitors numerous vital signs and runs dozens of tests throughout the surgery, continually adjusting the input of the machines to control the chemistry of the patient. Because these technologies now make it possible for the surgeon to fix complicated problems inside the narrow chambers of the heart, an attending doctor is necessary to pry the heart open and hold it in the correct position while the surgeon places his hands inside to repair it. Meanwhile, a scrub nurse juggles countless instruments and other pieces of equipment, handing the surgeon each in turn and helping prepare the bypass grafts. A minimum of five highly skilled professionals work constantly during each operation, every one of them responsible in different ways for whether the patient lives or dies. Depending upon the complexity of the operation, three to five more professionals may be necessary. The operating room is densely stacked with computer monitors, vials, tubes, lights, heating and cooling machines, and instruments of all kinds. But the better medicine gets at this type of surgery, the more people are needed to carry it out.

Because of remarkable improvements in its effectiveness

since the mid-1970s, coronary bypass surgery is now one of the most common operations: some 350,000 patients get it every year, more than double the rate ten years ago. Since recent studies indicate that patients in their eighties seem to survive this surgery about as well as people half their age, the aging of the population will probably increase the demand for such operations. Many patients will have two or three heart operations, including bypass and valve replacements, as advanced age brings more life-threatening malfunctions. The 150 or so hospitals currently performing heart transplants are likely to grow in number, and the volume of the surgery (currently more than 2,000 transplants a year) will increase.

Most patients survive these operations, largely because as soon as surgery is completed, they are whisked to an intensive care unit and hooked up to more banks of computerized monitors, diagnostic machines, and life-support equipment. Highly skilled doctors and nurses watch the monitors around the clock, adjusting the technological input and medications to carry the patient safely through this extremely fragile transition. Before the operation started, other specialized technicians operating high-tech diagnostic equipment mapped the problems that the surgeon was charged with repairing. Taken together, the absolute minimum number of skilled medical professionals required for the operations is about twenty-five, aided by another ten to twenty technicians and support personnel. As medicine has gotten better in this area, its productivity has declined.

There are exceptions to the Baumol phenomenon. Using the latest equipment, for example, doctors can perform simple lab tests in their offices that formerly took two to three days or had to be done by outside specialists. Results are available immediately, precise diagnosis takes less time, and theoretically more patients can be served efficiently. Most medical technology, though, yields smaller productivity gains while dramatically boosting the number of patients who seek its superior benefits.

To gain control of health spending, specific costs can be attacked. But short of denying medical care that doctors think people need, there would seem to be strict limits on just how sharply long-term medical cost inflation can be curbed. Unless, of course, medical research makes some quantum leaps that cannot yet be predicted with certainty. It has before.

8

SOMEONE ELSE'S MONEY

If you think health care's expensive now, wait until
it's free.
— Bumper sticker spotted by Richard Scott, CEO,
Columbia/HCA Healthcare

MORE than anything else, medical consumption is driven
by the fact that four out of five Americans, the rich as well
as the poor, buy their health care with someone else's
money. Health care is now viewed as a consumer good.
Americans have come to expect the best. Why shouldn't
they? Unlike buyers of any other consumer good, health
customers don't pay the bulk of the bill.

Typically, medicine today is paid for by some unseen insurance company, government agency, or other third-party
payer. This third party is not present when the doctor and
patient decide to spend health dollars but is instrumental to
the doctor-patient relationship. Whether covered under indemnity plans or managed-care plans, most privately insured Americans pay no more than about 20 percent of the
price. Similarly, by absorbing most or all of the costs of
many services, Medicaid and Medicare generate wasteful
consumer demand. Stanford economist Alain Enthoven
explains: "When you are insured, whether by private

companies or by the government, you do not have a serious, personal reason to care about health-care cost increases. You're buying it with somebody else's money. Your doctor doesn't have any reason to care about the cost increases, either, because insurance pays."

In that sense, insurance has long given doctors and hospitals the freedom to spend money however they saw fit. Insurance has also enabled medical research to advance rapidly, while fueling consumer demand for health services by ensuring payment of the bills. Blue Cross, the first of the big group plans, was started in Dallas in 1929 when Baylor University Hospital agreed to provide fifteen hundred local schoolteachers up to twenty-one days of hospital care per year for $6 apiece.[1] Baylor wanted to be sure its bills were paid, and group coverage was a way to guarantee it. Financially troubled hospitals soon embraced the idea and the plans proliferated. Several years later, Blue Shield was formed to cover physicians' services. By the middle 1930s, commercial insurers began covering hospitalization and surgery.

During World War II, corporations began offering employee insurance plans in large numbers when the government decided that moderate fringe benefits would not defeat the wartime price controls that were capping wages. Good workers were hard to find during wartime. Companies saw employee benefits as a way of attracting the best people, and health coverage was inexpensive. Once unions gained the right to bargain collectively for health benefits, medical coverage began to be perceived as a right, and companies were more firmly locked into offering it as a competitive weapon. Meanwhile, the Hill-Burton Act, passed in an effort to improve and modernize hospital facilities, had created a vast new stream of revenues for hospital construction. Between 1947 and 1971, $3.7 billion in taxpayer funds contributed to about a third of all hospital expansion.[2]

In 1965, the federal government became a major provider of insurance. President Lyndon Johnson signed the Medicare and Medicaid legislation, extending hospital and physician benefits to the poor, the elderly, and the disabled. Now that most Americans were insured, spending for medical services began to grow briskly.

Right from the start, the new federal guarantees of payment pumped up costs, making health care more expensive for everyone. The surge of public spending put a floor under prices and helped make medicine a "cost-plus" business. Whatever the doctors and hospitals charged, the government paid. As those higher prices were also demanded of the privately insured population, they pushed up commercial insurance premiums. The health sector now began to be described as "recession-resistant." The name stuck. No matter what was happening in the economy, health spending rocketed ahead of general inflation, and health employment grew.

> We cannot go on as we have in the past. New patterns will be necessary. Those who entertain some apprehension as to what the new patterns will be had better plunge in and experiment with their own preferred solutions. Standing back and condemning the solutions that others devise won't stem the tides of change.

That bold statement regarding the need for substantive health system reform was made in 1967 by John W. Gardner, President Johnson's Secretary of Health, Education and Welfare.[3]

When Gardner spoke up, the disturbing consequences of the first massive federal experiment in health insurance were becoming evident. The Medicare and Medicaid systems had been in place for less than two years, and costs were already rising far faster than anyone had projected. It turned out that in its attempt to solve the health needs of the poor, the elderly, and the disabled, the federal government had created a new form of currency — federal health dollars — that created peculiar distortions in the health market. If the government said it would pay for something, be it hospitalization or technology, a lot of that product or service was used and prices for the services rose.

In the case of Medicaid, the complicated federal rules helped to cripple the effectiveness of the program. Medicaid's requirements that many patients be hospitalized to receive care, for instance, were great for the hospitals. Treating large numbers of Medicaid patients was a way of attracting a lot of federal funding. Hospitals used the money to expand. Since these new public dollars were available in almost unlimited supply, there were none of the usual incentives to perform at a reasonable price. To make sure that hospitals treated Medicaid and Medicare patients, the original legislation paid them on a cost-plus basis, guaranteeing them a profit margin in addition to whatever they billed as costs. Guess what happened to costs? As the Health Policy Advisory Center, a small, nonprofit New York City think tank, put it in 1970:

> The peculiar thing about Medicaid money is that the more you spend, the less it's worth. In the first year of the Medicaid (and Medicare) program, doctors' fees rose 2.4 times as fast as the overall cost of living. Hospital costs rose four times as fast as the cost of living. A reasonable increase in hospital prices should have been expected in the late '60s, because of higher wages for nonprofessionals, the high costs of new life-saving equipment, etc. But costs never would have risen so high so fast without Medicaid and Medicare.[4]

Health providers were able to cross-subsidize their construction, training, technology, and other costs simply by billing the government more. Wall Street analysts touted hospital suppliers as a sure bet, and, for years, they were. By 1968, an unpleasantly surprised Congress began slashing Medicaid funds in order to control spending — but without curbing the misguided federal Medicaid rules that were driving the costs.

A brutal cycle ensued. The states were responsible for the majority of Medicaid costs, but the federal government still made most of the rules. The complex federal requirements made Medicaid expensive to provide. By cutting the federal funding, Congress put the states in a squeeze. The costs for treating individual patients were still going up, and the federal subsidies were going down. The only way that states could control their spending was to deny Medicaid benefits to people. They began to trim the rolls by tightening eligibility standards. By 1991, Medicaid was our fastest-growing spending program, a gas-guzzler dispensing $158 billion in federal and state funds to 27.3 million Americans. By 1993, 28.5 million Americans were on Medicaid.[5] But millions of other poor people who needed health services had been trimmed from the rolls. This voracious public-spending program, which cost $2.3 billion in its first year and today costs 70 times as much, now can afford to cover only 40 percent of America's poor.[6] Annual health costs for each Medicaid beneficiary are more than twice as high as for privately insured Americans.[7] The nursing-home industry has boomed, thanks to Medicaid funding. But the program designed for the poor has little left for most of them.

The well-meaning piece of legislation that Congress thought would improve care for the poor is partly responsible for the decline in the quality of medical care for many of the poor. Rural and inner-city residents who once had greater access to charity care, however degrading it may have seemed, now have less access in many cases to health services of any kind.

Medicaid, though, was merely an afterthought piece of legislation, an entitlement tacked on to the Medicare bill as a political compromise. Medicaid proponents had said it would cost only $1 billion by 1990 (actual 1990 costs: $76 billion). Medicare was the point of the effort. Political leaders agreed that America's pensioners had to be protected against medical costs and made the elderly a promise to provide coverage for medical care, never foreseeing the expansion of services that would ensue, or the demand. When Congress set up the program in 1965, the experts said that by 1990 Medicare would cost $9 billion. By 1990, though, the Medicare tab was running $70 billion per year, and by 1993 it was $128.8 billion. What happened? For one thing, medicine got a lot better at saving older people's lives. Retirees were visiting their parents in nursing homes.

More important, the Medicare entitlement took the financial pain out of health decisions. Medicare, for example, agreed to pay doctors the "usual and customary fees" for their services. Several years after the program was started, some of these fees were frozen in an attempt to curb double-digit inflation in Medicare spending. Doctors easily found a way around that problem. New treatments and procedures were coming on-line all the time; physicians began charging exorbitant fees for new treatments as a way of setting the "usual and customary" bar high. Example: gastroenterologists had been charging $50 to $60 for examining the colon with a proctoscope. When a new, slightly different scope became available, the gastroenterologists began charging $1,000 for the test.[8]

All in all, Medicare transformed the health-spending power of older Americans. In addition to giving them greater access to physicians and hospitals, it has helped make the selling of medical equipment and services to the elderly a booming business that will only grow. Guaranteed

Medicare financing of some costs has fostered impressive product innovation, and medical products for the elderly have taken on a consumer polish. One example: souped-up wheelchairs with heavy rear tires that enable people to get around when they can no longer drive a car. Assured payment has also given rise to plenty of excess and what can only be called consumer fraud. Some hospital employees have been accused of taking kickbacks to recommend equipment and services to departing Medicare patients. But even without the imprimatur of a hospital recommendation, elderly patients and their worried spouses are vulnerable to the aggressive marketing tactics of manufacturers of unnecessary high-cost items.

To many elderly consumers, a recommendation from the representative of a health manufacturer carries the aura of medical authority. The manufacturers often exploit that. In Los Angeles last year, for example, a sales representative for an exorbitantly priced special bed clinched one sale by assuring the patient's wife that Medicare would pay for part of it. She felt obliged to buy the $1,000 bed for her desperately ill husband, even though her daughter, a physician, told her that it would do nothing to help the father. "What could I do?" said the daughter. "She was determined. It wasn't about the bed; it was about loyalty and love." Since Medicare paid part, the price did not seem so high, and the worried wife followed her instinct to comfort her husband. The daughter helped pay for it, and, of course, so did Medicare. Thousands of decisions like that are made every day.

In 1983, trying to gain control over Medicare hospital costs, Congress tried price controls. It defined nearly five hundred types of hospital care called Diagnosis-Related Groups (DRGs) and set flat prices for each category. If hospitals treated a Medicare patient for less than the DRG rate, they made a profit. If not, they lost money. The price controls did not work as intended. Congress thought that the

controls would make hospitals more efficient, forcing them
to do everything for Medicare patients more cheaply. Instead, many hospitals responded by giving Medicare patients less care. As price controls always do, the DRGs
created a form of shortages. The shortage in this case was
time in the hospital. Many hospitals began releasing Medicare patients earlier than they should to save money. The
word "well" was redefined for elderly patients to mean: It's
time for you to go. Still, the hospitals figured they were losing anywhere from 10 percent to 20 percent on each Medicare patient they treated.

Meanwhile, in some cities, the price controls seemed to
change the doctor's diagnoses: suddenly more patients were
reported to be suffering from the forms of heart disease that
qualified for the highest DRG reimbursements. Before
DRGs, only 35 percent of Medicare patients in certain cities
were diagnosed with acute heart disease; after DRGs, doctors said that 48 percent of the patients had it. Before the
price controls were put in place, 64 percent of Medicare patients had the lower-cost chronic heart disease; afterward,
only 52 percent had it.[9] This was an example of "code
creep." Whether filling out Medicare papers or commercial
insurance forms, some doctors and hospitals have a tendency to exaggerate what they do for patients by choosing
an insurance identification code that describes a more expensive treatment. The heart patients had been "upcoded,"
or nudged into the higher category of reimbursement. "Unbundling" was another accounting trick that caught on in
hospitals. Instead of reporting some surgeries as a single
procedure, a physician or hospital would bill every step of
the operation as a separate job. It paid. A $2,900 gastrec-
tomy, which is the removal of part or all of the stomach,
could be billed a la carte as several different procedures for a
total of about $7,000. Unbundling was very similar to what

auto shops sometimes do when they charge several times for breaking down the engine to make repairs, when in fact they only broke down the engine once and did all of the repairs at the same time.

Doctors, nurses, and hospital administrators began to attend seminars in "creative accounting," a reference to the art of filling out insurance forms for maximum reimbursement. Some of these seminars were advertised openly in medical periodicals. Most health professionals did not consider the accounting practices particularly unethical. In their view, they were "playing Robin Hood." By defeating the arbitrary restrictions invented by bureaucrats, they argued, they were able to capture more reimbursement money, which they could then use for such laudable purposes as training more residents, improving the quality of their equipment, and providing more care to the indigent. And what about the fact that these practices were driving up medical prices and therefore raising everyone's insurance premiums? Hospital administrators glossed over the fact that in padding their bills, they were helping to make medicine as well as insurance too costly for some people to afford. Creative accounting became more widespread, and all insurance forms grew more complicated as insurers tried to fight back with more questions.

The forms have become the bane of patients' medical experience. They make everyone feel stupid and irritable. Financial or medical savvy have nothing to do with understanding them. Doctors and hospital administrators are often as mystified by them as anyone else. As chief executive officer of the New York Hospital and Cornell Medical Center, Dr. David Skinner is currently directing a $1 billion renovation and expansion of the sixty-year-old hospital. A master financial manager, he can juggle budget projections and turn them inside out with aplomb. But he sheepishly admits that he does not understand his own health insurance bills at all. When a visitor challenges him, assuming that he is joking, Dr. Skinner flushes with anger: "I'm telling you, I don't understand them." Neither does Dr. James Todd of the American Medical Association. He recalls his immense frustration trying to figure out the bills a couple of years ago when his father was dying. "Finally, I just had to give up. I stopped by my old office in New Jersey and threw myself on the mercy of one of the nurses there. She helped me figure them out."

President Clinton has aptly described the incomprehensible tangle of medical paperwork as "the Rube Goldberg system of payment." The paperwork can be seen as the devastating exchange of fire in the epic accounting wars that have broken out between providers and insurers, both the federal insurance plans and the commercial ones. Third-party payment started the war. Studies estimate that we spend about $100 billion per year filling out those forms. Each of the more than fifteen hundred different health insurance companies brandishes its own forms and procedures. Medicare and Medicaid rules read like the Encyclopedia Britannica.

Those who pay the medical bills wonder if the treatment was really needed and whether the price is right. They fight from afar with armies of accountants and blizzards of arcane rules that have nothing to do with helping people feel better. Those gleaming high-rise office towers that house the large insurance companies are filled with the clatter of calculators and the glow of computer screens as thousands of number crunchers try to figure out how to curb costs. The same activities go on in some of those massive government buildings in Washington. Meanwhile, just about every hospital devotes a floor to the files and clerks and computers.

Right in the middle of this accounting cross-fire are the

hard-working doctors and nurses who must spend precious hours filling out forms, employing arcane insurance codes to describe what they are doing for patients and why, often forced as a result of all this bureaucracy to forgo giving the patients attention that would make a real difference. In one small California hospital with fifty beds, two nurses work the night shift: one takes care of the patients, while the other one sits all night filling out insurance forms. Says the one who makes the rounds: "I've been a nurse for more than twenty years. I know that it makes a real difference to people if you have a moment to talk. But I don't have the time anymore."

Clearly the paper costs must be contained. Switching to electronic payment would help. Simplifying insurance rules and converting to standard forms would, too. Trouble is, the same new federal health plan that may require such sensible changes will bring its own new avalanche of paperwork.

Even if it were possible to eliminate the paper costs entirely, medical inflation would not be curbed. Cutting such administrative costs yields a one-time savings. Medical costs will still continue to rise because the essential dynamics of growth in health spending are medical progress, increasing demand, and guaranteed payment, or entitlement. Even as progress and demand are growing, we are about to gas up the entitlement engine. Entitlement creates excess demand because the illusion is created that the service is free. Third-party payment is the main reason health costs today are twenty-four times what they were in 1965 and the main reason that costs will continue to rise under any reform plan that guarantees coverage to everyone. It is one of the major obstacles threatening to defeat attempts to control spending while expanding that coverage. Giving all Americans a broad guarantee of coverage will create powerful new inflationary pressure. Only by crafting the new health system carefully will we be able to avoid losing control of health spending. In order to maintain some semblance of control, the natural restraining influence of personal responsibility must be built into the payment structure. Everyone must pay his or her share. In Alain Enthoven's words, each of us must have a "serious, personal reason" to care about health costs.

9

WHY DOCTORS, HOSPITALS, AND DRUGS COST SO MUCH

IF third-party payment is the recipe for higher costs, doctors, hospitals, and drugs are the main ingredients. Each contributes to the health bill in different ways, and until recently they all existed in a financial wonderland unlike the rest of the American economy, one where the prices usually were not questioned and often had little to do with the normal workings of supply and demand. All three parts of medicine are vital to the treatment of illness, and all have begun to temper their prices in the era of managed care.

Doctors are key to national health spending, since they make the decisions on patient care that result in nearly all health costs. They diagnose the patient, request the tests, hospitalize the sick, order and perform the surgery, and prescribe the drugs. And under the fee-for-service system that has long dominated American medicine, they have been paid separate fees for just about every single thing they did for patients.

Physician incomes always rise much faster than the

national inflation rate. In other occupations, an increasing supply of workers generally depresses prices, but not in medicine. There are twice as many physicians now as there were about twenty years ago. Taking population growth into account, that is about half again as many doctors per capita. If grocery store proprietors had multiplied as quickly, they would be having a hard time making ends meet. Yet what may look like a generous supply of doctors has done little to restrain physician incomes. Even though the physician's average number of weekly appointments with patients has declined during the past ten years, the average doctor's income after office expenses has risen by almost 70 percent, from $105,000 to $176,000. In 1992, the cost of an office visit for a new patient rose by 11 percent.[1] One change cushioning physician incomes: during the last thirty years, the cascading implications of medical research have driven doctors into many new medical occupations. Unable to master every aspect of modern medicine and eager to help develop medicine's growing knowledge of human illness and cures, doctors focused on parts of the human body and areas of study. The growing market supply of doctors divided itself into supplies of many kinds of doctors who were paid for doing different things.

Physicians typically believed they would be better doctors if they specialized. General practitioners were coming to be viewed by many of their colleagues as second-rate doctors, people who began to fall hopelessly behind the advance of knowledge the day they left school and began to practice. Kids smart enough to get into medical school thought they were aiming high by shunning family practice; they began to disdain family doctors. "They call them which doctors," says Dr. James Todd, executive vice president of the American Medical Association. "As in, 'I wonder which doctor I should send my patient to?' You can't blame these young people for not being motivated into that sort of sphere." And so as more and more physicians became more interested in medical science than in taking care of families, the family doctor began to disappear from many parts of the country. As doctors focused on narrower areas of study, whole new categories of special medical services were created. Instead of relying on family doctors to offer them guidance as to what they needed, more and more Americans began to find their way, ache by ache, through a costly specialized medical system.

Seven out of ten doctors are now specialists, and most medical students are planning to be. Well-insured American families have grown accustomed to having a whole deck of personal doctors — the internist, the gynecologist, the pediatrician, the urologist, the cardiologist — and to paying each of these specialists for examinations and tests. Doctors who specialize earn far higher incomes than family physicians. In 1992, cardiac surgeons made an average of $575,000, though some made more than $1 million; orthopedic surgeons averaged $339,829; anesthesiologists $253,511. Family physicians averaged $119,186; internists $129,787; pediatricians $123,870; gynecologists $173,884.[2]

The key difference in pay between a specialist and a family doctor is often that the specialist earns fees on a wider range of expensive tests and services. While the specialist can rack up enormous income in this piecework fashion, the family doctor essentially is paid for his or her time and has fewer opportunities to earn extra money by performing tests or specialized procedures. Specialists can argue quite persuasively, of course, that they deserve the higher pay, since the family doctor is often not capable of doing what they do. After all, what's a life worth?

But thirty years ago, the difference between the pay of specialists and family doctors was not nearly as great. It is primarily the method of payment that has created the differential and that has encouraged abuse. One of the worst consequences of the third-party payment system is the growth of fee-for-service medicine. Under this form of physician compensation, doctors earn more if they do more, regardless of the results for the patient. Research has shown that doctors paid in this manner order as many as 50 percent more electrocardiograms and 40 percent more X-rays than physicians in managed-care groups, who do not have the same financial incentives.

When doctors own labs and clinics and are in a position to send patients to them, the conflict of interest shows. The practice of prescribing treatments in facilities in which the physician holds a financial interest is called self-referral, and it is all too common. About 10 percent of U.S. physicians have investments in labs and other facilities to which they send patients. The problem is that they cannot make a profit on their investments unless the machines are heavily used. A Florida study found that doctors owned 93 percent of the diagnostic-imaging centers surveyed, 78 percent of the radiation-therapy centers, 60 percent of the clinical labs, and 38 percent of the physical therapy and rehabilitation centers. Miami doctors prescribed MRI scans twice as often as physicians in Baltimore, where very few own the equipment. Some investor groups setting up high-technology testing labs offer doctors limited partnerships, in which they make a small investment and are guaranteed a hefty return. The implication is that they will help keep those machines humming. In many cases, banks putting up the money for testing labs have required that physicians be included among the investors.

Even when the conflict of interest is not so clear, it can be exceedingly difficult to rule out the possibility that self-referrals are creating unnecessary usage. Physicians defend their role as investors and owners. After all, there is nothing wrong with making an honest profit — if that's what it is. They say that they are helping patients by coming up with the capital to buy the expensive technology that can dramatically improve their diagnostic skills. Doctors own most of the thirty MRI machines in Atlanta, and many send their patients to their own machines. In other states, many doctors own kidney-dialysis clinics and other outpatient treatment centers and are in a direct position to refer hospital patients for treatment.

The American Medical Association has condemned self-referral as unethical. But the practice has grown as hospitals have come under growing competitive pressure to cut costs. Federal regulations inadvertently encouraged self-referral through budget controls that pressured hospitals to cut short the hospital stays of some Medicare and Medicaid patients. Treatment was shifted to outpatient clinics. In many cases, physicians at the hospitals — or the hospitals themselves — captured the business by investing in the clinics, in part to make up for the income they were losing as Medicare and Medicaid limited their fees. In this way, some treatment costs were shifted off the hospital books, but the prices for overall treatment were not always reduced. In some cases, the cost of a given service rose.

When the federal government insisted on reducing costs in one category, doctors and hospitals found ways to shift them to another category. Providers won a skirmish in the accounting wars. Since 1992, a new law has forbidden doctors from referring Medicaid and Medicare patients to labs in which they have a financial interest. New York and Florida have banned some kinds of self-referrals. But the practice continues where it has not specifically been outlawed. Even in New York, doctors are still referring hospital patients to outpatient clinics in which the physicians have a financial interest.

HOSPITAL RATES

Americans spent more than $360 billion on their inefficient hospital system last year. That is more than $1,400 for every man, woman, and child in the country.

Are they getting their money's worth? Americans did not pay that much simply because they got so much care. They also paid for widespread inefficiency in hospitals, for astonishing waste, and for high salaries for hospital administrators and doctors, among other things. Hospitals operate in the same strange health economy as doctors and medical manufacturers. Medical prices reflect what the provider or manufacturer thinks the market will bear, but they also reflect administrative efficiency and professional quality. Because there is still little uniformity in medical practice standards or in insurance rates, prices in this peculiar industry bear no predictable relation to the actual costs of delivering the service. Nor are they always clearly related to the payment that is actually received for the service. A procedure that costs a doctor $50 to perform may be billed at $1,000 and reimbursed at $647 — or some other odd amount calculated in the insurer's accounting department.

Prices for the same treatment often vary dramatically and unpredictably within a given area. What, for example, should coronary bypass surgery cost? In her congressional testimony last fall, Hillary Rodham Clinton cited the case of three different Pennsylvania hospitals that charged prices for bypass surgery ranging from $21,000 to $84,000. She used the example to suggest that one hospital was unfairly getting several times as much money for exactly the same service. It looked that way. But she was mistaken.

In fact, the Pennsylvania example aptly illustrated the

deceptive nature of medical prices. While the three hospitals in question charged very different prices, they were actually paid almost the same amount for the operations. The Reading Hospital and Medical Center charged $21,063 for bypasses but received an average of $18,221 in insurance reimbursements. Meanwhile, the Graduate Hospital in Philadelphia charged $84,000, but was paid, on average, $23,974. Even though the Graduate's price was $63,000 higher than Reading's, the Graduate was actually paid only about $5,000 more for each of the operations. In most cases at the three hospitals cited, the bills were paid by Medicare and Medicaid, which have price controls, or else by large insurance companies, which have the clout to dismiss high prices like Graduate's and negotiate lower rates. Then why did the Graduate bother to charge $84,000? "Because there are still some people out there who will pay it," Samuel Steinberg, president of the Graduate, explained to a *Washington Post* reporter.[3] Some insurance companies will pay considerably more than others for certain procedures. And some patients, deciding where to have a crucial operation, will always think the higher-priced hospital must be the better one.

At one time, the prices more accurately reflected real costs, and the hospitals expected to be paid what they charged. During the last decade, though, the growing competition in medical care has forced hospitals to reexamine their practices and has driven down some hospital costs. As managed-care plans, the government programs, and insurers have brought pressure on the bills, hospitals have begun to question whether patients gain by spending so many days in them and have undertaken a broad analysis of the way they work in search of savings. Most American hospitals are not-for-profit institutions, but that is slowly changing. Much of the credit for the small gains that hospitals have made in efficiency belongs to the growing numbers of profit-making hospitals that began to compete for the right to serve patients.

Profit-making hospitals have introduced impressive management techniques to an industry that had never learned how to order supplies or organize its other functions any more efficiently than the Pentagon. The superior management systems are catching on, though they still have a long way to go. In the past, for example, patients routinely were kept in the hospital unnecessarily over the weekend simply because their doctors had not checked their condition in time to give them a green light before taking off on Friday. That was just fine with the hospitals, of course; they earned money by keeping the beds occupied over the weekend. Now most doctors and hospitals must be more disciplined. Similarly, patients were often told to check in on Sunday for Monday surgery, adding one more day to the bill. Hospitals have learned to instruct the patient carefully on dietary requirements the day before surgery and to perform presurgery tests on an outpatient basis, in order to eliminate the need for many patients to check in early.

In the more wasteful era just a few years ago, hospitals knew and cared nothing about "discharge planning," a reference to the coordination of preparations to release patients to go home. Very often, patients had to stay an extra day because no one bothered to tell their families to come pick them up, or ordered that final laboratory test that would verify that they were well enough to go home. The people who made the discharge decisions did not coordinate with the people who treated the patients.

Hospitals were famous for having warehouses filled to the rafters with supplies of all kinds because no one was managing the inventory properly. Hospital administrators made little or no effort to buy in volume at discount. Usually, they had no incentive to do so; someone would pay. Similarly, new technology was ordered in haphazard ways. A medical-devices salesman would sweep through a hospital, demonstrate a new gadget, and book sales. Doctors would then start using the gadget to find out how well it worked. Administrative functions were needlessly duplicated in different departments, which were allowed to defend their autonomy within the institution regardless of the waste it generated. As not-for-profits, most hospitals did not have to perform efficiently, especially in the era when insurers were passive about paying bills. If the hospitals came out ahead, they spent it, usually by adding services, space, or technology. In forming its new network, New York Hospital saved more than $1 million a year simply by consolidating a few administrative departments.

Now that they are under greater cost pressure, hospitals are beginning to correct the old mindless practices. But inefficiency persists, since most hospitals still do not have to make a profit. Because hospitals still get paid much like hotels, by the number of days that people stay in them, many hospital administrators stay up nights trying to figure out how to put more paying patients in the beds. One way to do so is by loading up on the latest high technology so that they can offer new medical services. Other hospitals, of course, are thinking the same thing. And so for no good reason, hospitals a block or two apart buy the same MRI machines, and those hospital administrators are staying up nights all over again trying to figure out how to amortize the costs of the new equipment by making sure that people in the area use their machines, not their competitor's. One typical answer: hire more specialists and build up that part of the business. A heart surgeon can bring in millions of dollars a year; a large cardiothoracic practice can be a gold mine. Theoretically, a single heart patient may at different times need angioplasty, in which a tube inserted into an artery pushes a blockage out of the way (at a cost upward of $15,000); a bypass or two ($40,000); a heart valve replacement ($50,000); and eventually a heart transplant (at least $100,000). Earning prestige in such areas of medical practice builds the reputation of the institution and attracts patients who need other kinds of service and believe that the hospital is superior in all ways.

Since different kinds of insurance pay different rates, part of the job of hospital administrators is to make sure their institutions attract enough patients who will pay more. Rich patients often make generous endowments as well. In New York City, Columbia Presbyterian has a gourmet service for rich patients, complete with private sitting rooms and other amenities. The idea is to charge them more and use the money to fund things like indigent care, research, and other expenses — including the salaries of the top specialists who bring in many of those well-heeled patients. Across town, New York Hospital, a leading teaching institution, says it is working with the Four Seasons restaurant to see if it can make its food a lot tastier.

Hospitals began to become accountable for their costs when insurers (including employers who self-insure) started aggressively questioning bills and investor-owned hospitals began to compete for the business. Because the nonprofits were so wasteful, the investor-owned hospitals knew that even in an era of belt-tightening, they could carve out a piece of the business, operate more efficiently than the competition, and make a profit. The nonprofits had produced too many wings and too many hospital beds and hired all the people they needed to run the place as if it were full. Currently, on any given day, one-third of all U.S. hospital beds are unoccupied. Stated in industrial terms, America has about one-third too much hospital capacity.[4]

As insurers continue to crack down on unnecessary tests, surgeries, and days in the hospital, it is getting harder for hospital administrators to balance their books by filling the beds.

The investor-owned hospitals have begun to transform the industry by introducing businesslike practices that seemed alien at first. The idea of closing down underused hospitals, for example, was once anathema. Hospitals had come to be viewed as community assets and sources of jobs. Communities and urban neighborhoods counted on third-party payers to keep their local hospitals open, no matter how inefficient or unnecessary the institutions might be. That has changed. Columbia / HCA Healthcare, for instance, is now the largest American hospital company. Columbia has often added market share by targeting cities that have too many underused hospitals. The firm buys up two or three of the hospitals, closes one of them, and combines the operations in the remaining facilities. Overnight, the Columbia hospitals become more efficient.

Another practice popularized by some investor-owned hospitals is giving doctors a piece of the business. Physicians affiliated with these institutions become part-owners, which may sometimes give them an incentive to refer more of their patients to the profit-making institution in which they have an interest. The white coat covers a pin-striped suit.

That is what is so disturbing to many people about the growing trend of hospitals and health plans buying physician practices. What exactly are they buying? The relationship of trust with the patient? The implication is that the doctors will feed patients to the business. The danger is that they might sometimes be inclined to order questionable treatment, particularly if they stand to earn a significant fraction of their incomes by doing so. In California and other states, some sales of physician practices to hospitals and health firms have been investigated as possible insurance fraud, on the theory that if improper financial incentives lead doctors to prescribe unnecessary medical care, the insurer who pays for it has been defrauded. Generally, the practice sales are considered to be acceptable if the physician leaves the practice or retires within about a year. The rationale: the doctor is not staying around to refer patients to the hospital. Even so, the suggestion lingers that these physicians have sold the relationship of trust with their patients. The sale price can be viewed as the departing physician's "golden parachute."

While the investor-owned hospitals have helped spur the industry toward more sensible management and greater efficiency, that does not mean their prices are always lower than those at the nonprofits. As investor-owned firms, they are motivated to build market share and earn profits. At times, when for-profit companies enter a hospital market, some prices increase as they begin engaging in aggressive marketing and complex pricing strategies. Some for-profit hospitals follow the time-honored retail practice, familiar to department store shoppers, of "marking it up in order to mark it down." They set their prices a bit high, then offer big discounts to employers or other representatives of large groups of potential patients, such as HMOs. In retail terms, these hospitals hold a private sale for preferred customers. Like retailers, they are counting on unsophisticated consumers to buy on the discount, rather than the actual charge. A better hospital nearby may charge a lower price than the for-profit hospital's discounted rate, but the buyer will never check. Chances are, the buyer or individual patients will be distracted by the for-profit hospital's nice receptionist, handsome decor, and great parking, and think they are getting a deal. Meanwhile, the surgeons at the cheaper hospital may be demonstrably superior. Until the public has access to better and more reliable information about the relative quality of the medical services offered by doctors, hospitals, and health plans, the prices they charge will continue to offer a poor yardstick by which to measure them.

DRUGS: A LITTLE PILL FOR EVERY ILL

What is a prescription for heart medicine worth? The pharmacy two blocks from your home may charge twice as much as the drugstore a mile in the other direction, and both may charge far more for the pills than the HMO down the road. Explanations for these price differentials vary. The lower-cost pharmacy may be part of a chain that gets volume discounts from the manufacturer, just as Macy's gets discounts on socks. Same medicine, very different price. The average prescription cost in the United States is $25,[5] but tell that to the patient who just paid $5 a pill. Most people who need prescription drugs are unhappy with prices, mainly because Americans pay, on average, 75 percent of the cost out of their own pockets. Drugs are the only part of health care where anyone has a sense of the real costs. And because drugs are a form of medical therapy, people are often surprised to find that prices can vary from store to store.

The cost of drugs must be judged in part, of course, by the savings they make possible in health and productivity. Research pharmaceuticals have conquered countless diseases and disabling conditions. They control heart disease, diabetes, and other chronic life-threatening ailments. Just one Merck drug, Vasotec, when added to previously used drug treatment for chronic heart failure, reduced the risk of death by 18 percent and the need for hospitalization by 30 percent, according to a five-year study sponsored by the National Heart, Lung and Blood Institute. The study concluded that the drug could prevent 20,000 deaths and save 100,000 hospitalizations every year. Estimated annual savings: $1 billion.[6] Other drugs enable schizophrenics, depressives, and other mentally ill Americans to live fairly normal lives. Clozaril, from the Sandoz company, makes it possible for many hospitalized schizophrenics to go home. One study showed that annual hospital bills dropped from $44,810 to $2,592 for patients who began to use the drug.[7] Similarly, a study showed that an asthma medication for a child that cost $431 a year eliminated 96 percent of trips to the emergency room and 62 percent of hospitalizations. Savings: $2,250.[8]

Drugs save babies born with defects that otherwise would kill them. They interrupt catastrophic injury by regulating the body's chemistry during trauma, giving doctors time to repair the damage. They also help save millions of lives every year by making complex operations possible, controlling the myriad internal functions of the patient during surgery's violent disruption of normalcy. They dissolve heart blockages, kill cancer cells, and stimulate the body to create healthy new cells after it is horribly damaged by burns. They clear up ulcers and infections and alleviate pain.

"What do you want when something is very wrong with you?" asks Dr. Charles Sanders, a cardiologist who is chairman of the Glaxo pharmaceutical company. "You want a little pill to make you better."[9] Sanders should know: Glaxo makes Zantac, the ulcer medication that is one of the world's best-selling drugs — and has helped make ulcer surgery all but obsolete. During the next twenty years, researchers anticipate that advances in drug therapies will save $76 billion in Alzheimer's treatment and $12 billion for arthritis care.[10] According to William Steere, Jr., the chairman of Pfizer, "Our companies are the future of health-care cost containment."[11]

The pharmaceutical business is a relatively small part of

the health sector, but it is growing fast. In 1992, revenues totaled $76 billion; 1993 sales were expected to reach $85 billion. The aging of the population is slowly creating a boom market for drugs that can control chronic disease and replace surgery or hospitalization. And if national health reform extends prescription drug coverage to all Americans, that will mean more than 72 million new insured customers for the drug companies. Because of its success in formulating new therapies, the pharmaceutical industry is already one of the strongest export sectors. Federal economists say that it is the only major American export industry that did not lose ground during the 1980s. If *The Graduate* were made today, one could imagine the businessman sidling up to Dustin Hoffman and muttering, "Valium."

But do the drugs cost too much? The Clinton administration says they do, and in some cases, the prices are astonishing. The current wholesale price for one patient's annual supply of Clozaril is about $4,000. Some people would call that a fair trade, considering that it saves more than $40,000 in annual hospital costs; others call it price-gouging. Centocor priced Centoxin, a promising treatment for often-fatal septic shock, at more than $3,000 for each dose during its initial marketing. Negative test results shot down the drug, but not before the price set off a wave of outrage.

Critics of drug companies point out that manufacturing costs for drugs are often no more than a fraction of a cent a pill or liquid dose, which then may sell for several dollars. Drug companies riposte that it is not their manufacturing expenses, but the intellectual costs of bringing these miracle pills to market that are so high.

Drugs are products. Their price reflects not only the simple chemical content of a medicine and the costs of making it, but also the costs of research, marketing, testing, borrowing capital, and putting aside profits. In 1992, the pharmaceutical industry spent $12.5 billion on research and development. These days, the Pharmaceutical Manufacturers Association estimates that it costs $270 million to bring a new drug to market.

Pharmaceutical firms are now investing in additional labs and testing facilities to explore the astonishing potential of the new field of biotechnology. In biotech, scientists alter the genetic structure of animals and plants to create new characteristics or to fix flaws. In its simplest form, biotechnology can change fruits and vegetables to make them more resistant to harsh weather or insects. But looming directly ahead is the possibility that medical scientists will be able to make small changes in human genes to prevent diseases from developing. Already, scientists have identified the genes at fault for several major ills, including cystic fibrosis, sickle cell anemia, Down's syndrome, hemophilia, muscular dystrophy, Huntington's disease, "Lou Gehrig's disease" (amyotrophic lateral sclerosis), the "bubble-boy" syndrome, a common form of colon cancer, one type of Alzheimer's, and the nerve disease portrayed in the film *Lorenzo's Oil,* and they are close to pinpointing the location of the breast cancer gene.[12] The next step is to learn how to repair those genes. Biotech may hold the cures. As Dr. Richard Weinshilboum, vice chair of the Mayo Clinic board of trustees, puts it: "The field is developing very quickly. In five or ten years, you may not need a pill for Alzheimer's. We'll just fix the Alzheimer's gene. Before long, instead of doing open-heart surgery, we may be able to prevent a gene from expressing itself as coronary disease."[13]

The possibilities for new pharmaceutical products are remarkable. But no matter how significant a new medication may be, inventing it gives a company only a limited period of time to profit handsomely from ownership of the process. When pharmaceutical companies invent a new medicine, their patent runs out seventeen years after the discovery, but often only about ten years after they finally succeed in developing and testing the drug and bringing it to market. Once the patent expires, makers of generic drugs can start selling copies and capturing market share. The research pharmaceutical companies argue that they have to charge more for their medicines because they have a limited time to recover their investment costs. Moreover, once the patent runs out, market share can drop precipitously: managed-care firms often stipulate that they will not pay for a brand-name pharmaceutical if a cheaper generic version is available. About half of all prescription drugs dispensed in the United States are now subject to similar managed-care restrictions; generics account for close to a third of prescription drug sales.[14] Sure, generics are usually cheaper, the research drugmakers say; the $22 billion generics industry sells off-brand versions of medicines that other companies have spent a lot of money to invent. The pharmaceutical manufacturers also point out that, like oil men, they drill a lot of dry holes looking for new winners.

All of these defenses are valid as far as they go, but they are far from the whole story. Drug companies are the beneficiaries of federal research: they don't always have to spend a lot to develop a new product. And once in a while, they're just plain lucky. In 1992, after a Mayo Clinic physician discovered that a common sheep medication (price: $14) was effective in treating colon cancer, Johnson and Johnson began selling Ergamisol, the new version of the drug developed for humans, for $1,300 a dose. A 1991 Senate report called attention to some enormous price increases for prescription drugs that are hard to explain away as the cost of research. Wyeth-Ayerst, for example, raised the price of Premarin, an estrogen replacement, by 131 percent between 1985 and 1990; its Inderal heart medication went up 112 percent during the same period, while the Consumer Price Index was rising by only 21 percent. The calming and sleep-inducing medication Halcion, from Upjohn, more than doubled in price between 1985 and 1991, according to another study, while McNeils's Tylenol with codeine rose by 160 percent.[15]

There's nothing illegal about high prices, of course. But drugs are different from other products: often there is only one that will truly make a difference. Drug manufacturers have long had an extraordinary advantage in keeping their prices comfortably high: prescription drugs were ordered exclusively by doctors. Only the doctors had to be sold. Through prescriptions, they effectively created market share for drugs. If a new drug was only slightly different from an existing medication, but the doctor believed that the tiny difference was important to patients, the new drug could take the market away.

For years doctors have learned much of what they know about new drugs from "detail men," those well-compensated pharmaceutical salesmen who would breeze by, bringing literature and free samples. Like any other sales organization courting key clients, the drug companies have always been generous to physicians. Some hosted parties and outings for doctors and medical students that rivaled the lavish recruiting rituals of Wall Street firms and movie companies. "Come on down to Cancun," they'd say, "and learn about our great new medicine. We'll pay." And then there was Drug Day.

Jack Lewin will never forget his first exposure to Drug Day at the University of Southern California. It was 1967, and he was a first-year student at the medical school. Every month, all of the big pharmaceutical companies would put on a sort of drug fair for the medical students in an enormous auditorium. "It was just like the circus," he recalls, "or the auto show. There was a raucous party atmosphere. Each company had its own booth. There were women walking around in bathing suits. You wouldn't believe it! They'd sashay around and greet these work-crazed medical students and invite them to take free samples. They were giving away pens, and shirts, and chances for free trips to Hawaii and stuff. They actually gave away diet pills containing amphetamines — they said they'd help us study — and Valium and all kinds of other controlled substances. The medical students went from booth to booth with shopping bags, collecting all of these free drugs." Lewin remembers, "I came from a good, solid middle-class background in Orange County. I wasn't radical. I wasn't even really against the Vietnam War. I just didn't think this was right. I had just read an article by the head of the Food and Drug Administration that said that half the cost of drugs for senior citizens was to pay for physician advertising, promotions, and giveaways."

The following month, when Drug Day rolled around, Jack Lewin was there — with his own table, right at the main entrance. "I made a huge poster. I listed all the brand-name drugs and the names of the companies that made them on one side, with their prices. On the other side, I listed the generic equivalents with their prices. I put it up where it was the first thing you saw as you entered the room. You absolutely couldn't miss it. I was handing out information telling medical students that it was their duty to prescribe generics whenever possible."

The pharmaceutical representatives objected. They told him he had to leave. Lewin refused. Finally, they called the police and had him arrested. Lewin sat in the cell, wondering how much trouble he was really in and wondering why.

Later that evening Lewin said, a policeman came and let him out. "Roger Egeberg, the dean of the USC medical school, had heard about it and had come down to get me. He was like a god to us students. There he was, six foot five, standing there in a tuxedo. I thought he was going to give me hell. But he didn't. He got the charges dropped. He said I was doing what doctors should do, putting the interests of the patients first. He told me he was proud of me. I'll never forget him for that." Lewin got his medical degree. He now heads up Hawaii's pioneering health-care system, which since 1974 has provided low-cost health coverage to nearly all of its people. He is also a health adviser to President Clinton. He says he is a great admirer of pharmaceutical firms: "Their products are remarkable. As a doctor, I'd be lost without them. And the companies are a vital part of the American economy. It was Drug Day I couldn't abide."[16]

Extravaganzas like the one that got Lewin thrown in jail no longer take place, but Drug Day hasn't died out. It has only taken on a somewhat more subdued, educational mien. Last summer, in the surgical wing of a New York City hospital, a large, handwritten sign urged all to attend the annual deep-sea fishing trip sponsored by a pharmaceutical firm. (Drug Day goes to sea.) The price of admission: a conscience-salving $10, hardly enough to cover the expense. As recently as 1992, the *New England Journal of Medicine* published a series of letters from doctors debating the propriety of the sales techniques these companies still employ. Says one young Chicago physician of her first encounter during the 1980s with Drug Day: "I couldn't believe it. I thought it was insulting. You'd think we were a captive audience. Maybe we are."

Under managed care, fewer and fewer are. Many HMOs and hospitals now forbid detail men from visiting their physicians. Some draw up lists of approved drugs for their doctors, balancing effectiveness against price, and lock out the more expensive competitors. Like vendors in other industries, drug companies make discount deals with hospital and pharmacy chains. The pressure on drug prices is growing. If national reform adds coverage of prescription drugs for the elderly, the legislation will probably require selection of the lowest-priced alternative.

Looking for an edge, the drug companies have begun

wooing consumers directly. Since 1992, they have shifted much of their advertising from medical journals to mass-media periodicals. They are also beginning to engage in unprecedented marketing wars. In November 1993, Smith-Kline Beecham shook up the market by offering cash rebates to purchasers of the ulcer drug Tagamet, promising to save $20 a month off the cost of Zantac, its principal competitor. (In 1992 Tagamet sales were $1.1 billion; Zantac's were $3.5 billion.) SmithKline was under special pressure to build market share: once Tagamet's patent protection expires in 1994, competing generic versions will appear. That will put pressure on Zantac too. At the end of 1993, Upjohn was offering consumers coupons worth $30 off the price of Rogaine, a hair-replacement drug that retails for about $300, while Procter and Gamble, reaching all the way back to the 1960s for a promotional idea, introduced a money-back guarantee to patients who were not happy with Macrodantin and Macrobid, treatments for urinary tract infections.[17]

Meanwhile, the pharmaceutical firms still find other ways to keep their names uppermost in the minds of those in a position to prescribe. They sponsor medical conventions at which important research is presented. Critics say this is a form of advertising, but researchers and physicians (including Dr. Lewin) maintain that the meetings often make valuable contributions to the profession. On a more mundane level, the companies supply the handy pens, notepads, and other paraphernalia in doctors' offices and hospitals that carry pharmaceutical logos. In some hospitals, for example, nurses wear personal identification badges with a drug company's name discreetly printed in the corner. Unasyn gives away heavy-duty safety pins with its name on them so that surgeons and nurses, who cannot take any personal belongings into the operating room, can pin their locker keys to their scrubs. Doctors carry clipboards with a small drug company logo on the clamp.

To this day, physicians in private practice give patients the free samples delivered to them by eager salesmen. On the face of it, there would seem to be nothing wrong with this. "Except," says one doctor, "there's a subtle, corrosive aspect to it. You're busy. Maybe there are five or six different medications you could prescribe, and all of them work about as well. Maybe you prescribe one from a company that gave you free samples. It's familiar to you. You have seen it help your patients. Maybe it costs a little more than the others. You don't know. You're not buying it."

The forces driving up U.S. health costs cannot be contained simply by curbing prices, discouraging greed, and eliminating egregious bureaucracy and waste, though doing all of those things is critical. As American medical knowledge and our health needs grow, careful management of treatment resources will be the only way to ensure excellence. The alternative is unnecessary rationing of care if health funds cannot keep pace with medical need.

Already, the battle to control costs is constant and brutal, according to Dr. Brent James, executive director of the Institute for Health Care Delivery Research at Intermountain Health Care, a twenty-four-hospital chain headquartered in Salt Lake City. Intermountain's main hospital charges some of the lowest prices in the country for treating Medicare patients, after accounting for local cost of living and other factors. Yet even as it continually reduces the costs of caring for individual patients, its overall costs keep rising. James explains: "Our per-case costs are not growing. Actually, they are dropping. They're coming down 1 percent to 3 percent per year. But what we're finding is that no matter what we do, those gains are completely washed away by two other factors: new therapies that we simply did not do before and the important new technologies that come on the market.

That increases our overall costs by 3 percent or 4 percent, and eats up all of our savings. The other thing we're seeing is increasing demand for medical services as the population ages. Slowing the growth in spending is getting more difficult all the time."[18]

In all likelihood, it will only get harder.

10

THE BEAN COUNTERS: INSURANCE AND MANAGED CARE

ANY national health-reform law is likely to place a great emphasis on managed care and cost controls. Insurance companies and managed-care firms are best positioned to profit from such a restructuring of the national market, particularly if the law specifies a managed-competition system. Generally, health spending is slowed in two ways: by reducing access to health services or by limiting the money available to pay for care. Health maintenance organizations are expert in the first method: tightening up on care. Insurance companies try to use a little of both approaches. Ironically, insurers and HMOs are often two sides of the same company. Some managed-care plans, like Kaiser, provide their own insurance; many others, like Prudential's PruCare HMO, are owned by large insurance companies.

Of all the players in health care, none are viewed by the average person with as much hostility as the commercial insurance companies. More than a few public health officials, as well as some Clinton administration workers, would like to put them out of business altogether. People hate the insurance paperwork and resent the notion of a third wheel taking profit from the doctor-patient relationship. They wonder why there needs to be a profit-making company serving as middleman between the doctor and patient. One internist said: "Lawyers charge by the hour, and most of us family doctors do, too. But you don't pay a legal insurance company; you pay the lawyer. So why shouldn't people just pay the doctor directly?"

For one thing, medical care costs far too much. You never know when you will visit your doctor and tumble through the looking glass into that other realm of desperate illness and unbelievable expense. When one seemingly healthy and fit magazine editor went to his Manhattan dentist for a routine appointment in late 1992, he passed out as soon as the dentist tilted back the chair. That is how he learned he had a fast-growing brain tumor at the back of his head; the slight pressure produced by leaning back in the chair had triggered a reaction of distress in his injured brain. At work the next day, he joked about the blinding speed with which his entire future had been engulfed by medical distress. A few weeks later, he had brain surgery. Complications followed, and a long stretch in intensive care. Within six months after that unsuspecting visit to the dentist, he died. The bills were enormous. If not for his superior insurance coverage, his family would have been ruined.

Insurance used to be something everyone took for granted. But during the last ten years, health insurance premiums have mounted precipitously, making it impossible for many individuals and small companies to buy coverage. Americans have become all too familiar with the sinister term "preexisting conditions," which identifies medical problems incurred before the coverage took effect and for which the companies will not pay. Every day, it seems, they hear horror stories about people who were dropped by their insurers because they became seriously ill. What is insurance for, anyway, if they can drop you when you get sick? Are they that greedy?

Insurance is a balancing act called "risk management," but in recent years many health insurers have lost their balance. The key in risk management is to figure out the anticipated costs of health care for everyone in the group, from the sickest and oldest to the youngest and healthiest, then calculate average premiums to cover the expenses. All things being equal, covering 10,000 people is always cheaper than covering 500 people. Most people are healthy. The insurer is able to spread the risk, and the sickest people get the best value for their premium dollars. For-profit insurance firms add a small margin for their stockholders. Despite their evil reputations, though, commercial health insurance companies have averaged profits of less than 2 percent for more than ten years.[1] In other businesses, that kind of profit performance would get the chief executive fired. By comparison, hospitals make average profits (or, in not-for-profit parlance, "excess revenues") of 5 percent to 6 percent.[2] They earn three times the profit but nowhere near the enmity. Moreover, many nonprofit insurers, like regional Blue Cross/Blue Shield companies, have been in much worse financial trouble than the commercial companies and have raised their premiums far more abruptly. Several of these large nonprofit insurers have gone bankrupt, leaving their beneficiaries without coverage.

What happened? Until about ten years ago, risk management was made somewhat easier by the fact that most health insurance companies could count on covering large and diverse pools of people. But during the 1980s, as employers began to worry about rapidly rising health costs, many of them began to save money by self-insuring, cutting out the insurance company and setting up their own coverage for their workers. This was often cheaper, not least because employees of large companies tend to be healthier than the average population. There are no elderly, and most of the very sick do not hold full-time jobs with health benefits. Employers also liked self-insurance because very few state regulations covered such arrangements, and so they were often able to manipulate the finances and the rules to suit themselves. Many Americans who learned only when they became seriously ill that they were not covered blamed insurance companies for cold-hearted practices, never knowing that, in fact, it was their own employers who had made the stingy rules. One result of the self-insurance trend was that the insurance companies often found that they were left covering sicker and sicker people on average as self-insured groups of healthy people left their pools.

Equally important was the growth of HMOs and other managed-care plans. Younger and healthier people preferred the less-expensive managed-care plans because they did not need much health care, and most of what they did need was preventive care that had not been covered adequately under indemnity insurance. Meanwhile, older and sicker people with more complex medical needs preferred indemnity plans, which let them choose the doctors and health services they wanted. Many insurance plans thus suffered from "adverse selection," the tendency for sicker people to gravitate toward more generous plans and unbalance the budget. Some of those plans went down in flames as they entered what insurers call "the death spiral," an irreversible overload of sick beneficiaries that makes it impossible for premiums to keep up with costs.

As risk management in health became more difficult, some insurance companies competed by "cherry-picking," trying to choose only the healthiest, and therefore least expensive, groups to cover. They were able to do so because those groups, who were often workers at big companies that had not self-insured, liked the lower premiums they were offered. Cherry-pickers — including some big HMOs — sometimes cut corners on quality, figuring that anyone sick enough to care was a customer they did not want anyway. Because of these changes, small businesses and individuals began to be hit with exorbitant health insurance premiums. At a time when health costs were exploding, small businesses and families were not getting the cost advantage of sharing their financial health risk over a large group. Since most of the twenty million or so jobs created during the Reagan Miracle were small businesses and entrepreneurial shops, the trend was toward a more and more splintered insurance market: precisely what drives up premiums.

At the same time, many insurance companies were getting stuck with ill-advised investments in real estate that were going sour at a tremendous rate. They had invested in the commercial real estate boom of the 1980s that was pushed along by the corrupt and irresponsible savings and loan industry; when the S&Ls came apart, the commercial real estate markets dropped. Downtown high-rises were standing empty; out in the suburbs, shopping malls were left half completed. The tax reform legislation of 1986 worsened things by restricting the tax advantages of investing in real estate.

Since insurance companies rely on investment income to alleviate premium costs, the sudden real estate slump began to push up their premiums; insurers began to bear down harder on the health risk they were carrying. Company and family policies were canceled abruptly, sometimes when just one person contracted a serious illness. No one could believe this was happening. Insurance was supposed to be reliable. In 1992, one small but immensely profitable entertainment company in Beverly Hills was astounded when its coverage was canceled: one employee had contracted AIDS, and from the insurer's point of view, suddenly the risk of covering the other healthy and highly paid workers had skyrocketed. (An AIDS patient can incur as much as $1 million in medical costs.)

Everywhere in the United States this kind of insurance distress began to hit home. During the 1980s, some companies saw their premiums rise by 30 percent per year. Meanwhile, hidden in all that fine print that nobody ever read were a growing number of "exclusions," medical conditions that the insurer (or the self-insured corporation) refused to cover. Most people, of course, have no idea what their insurance policy says. They listen to the salesman or the company benefits representative and their eyes glaze over. Not until they get to the hospital do they learn that they are not covered for something they need right now. Doctors and hospitals hate the insurance companies as much as any worried family does. "They always make us tell people the bad news," says one doctor. Nobody reads the fine print until it is too late.

In mid-1992, the health insurance industry decided that things had gotten too far out of hand. The Health Insurance Association of America (HIAA) presented its agenda for national health reform: universal coverage; everyone would have the same benefits, and the benefits would be portable, meaning that people would not lose them if they changed jobs; insurers would levy reasonable premiums based on very large groups. No more preexisting-condition nonsense; no more excessive exclusions, and no more cherry-picking. Presidential candidate Bill Clinton applauded the suggestions as progressive. They sounded a lot like his own ideas. Health insurers contributed gladly to his campaign.

But once President Clinton got into the White House, he changed his public stance toward insurers. Administration officials began to castigate the insurance companies as heartless and profit-mongering. Speaking before a group of physicians, Hillary Rodham Clinton went so far as to say that insurance companies enjoyed dropping people's coverage because then they could make more money. Said Bill Gradison, a former congressman who now heads the HIAA: "The Clinton administration has described us as profiteering, cold-blooded, irresponsible, price-gouging, overcharging, and in other such warm and generous terms. I know we make an easy scapegoat, but they're wrong on the facts. We are for reform. We want to get everyone covered at an affordable cost. We don't want to cancel people, and we've been on record on that since Bush was president."[3]

So why don't they do it? They say that they need national reform as a framework so that everyone in their business will be playing by the same rules. What the insurance companies want is approximately what Bill Clinton has endorsed: some form of managed competition. Ironically, they see the national evolution toward managed care that caused them so much grief as the way out of trouble. The main reason is that so many insurers have given up their passive bill-paying role and have entered the managed-care industry. They are ready to compete for the business that the new health alliances would control.

Managed care now represents more than 60 percent of commercial insurers' group coverage business; their HMOs cover more than one-fifth of the U.S. subscriber total.[4] Aetna, for one, operates twenty-six HMOs, covering 1.2 million members.[5] The Prudential, Metropolitan Life, and other big companies are busily building up their own networks.

If everyone had to join health alliances, the insurance and health services market would rearrange itself rapidly into sprawling regional chunks. Big players, such as large HMOs, hospital chains, physician groups, pharmacy chains, and mail-order drug sellers like AARP, would be well positioned to capture much of the business before smaller competitors could organize themselves. The large insurance companies would win in at least two ways. Not only do they already run fast-growing HMO networks, but because of the favorable prices the alliances would offer people who chose managed-care plans, most of the insurance companies' current indemnity clients would probably be switching into something like HMOs. Since the companies are established in managed care, they would probably have the inside track as familiar name-brand providers when their indemnity clients shopped around. Moreover, managing the tightly constrained finances of the huge new health alliances described in the Clinton plan would be a daunting task; the large insurers have the most experience in managing risk. They say that if everyone in the country were under roughly the same kind of equitable insurance plan, they could profit by competing for customers on ye olde level playing field. But on this field, they are the Dallas Cowboys, and by comparison, most of the other players are from the Pee Wee League.

HMOs are the dominant model in managed care. They control costs by providing the full range of health services for a pre-set fee. In theory, they cut expenses by reducing waste. But until recently, they have not consistently performed better than indemnity insurance plans in terms of their price increases. They did not have to, so long as the costs of indemnity plans were out of control. The original HMO legislation allowed the plans to peg their prices to conventional insurance premiums. Many HMOs chose to engage in so-called shadow pricing to maximize their profits. They started out offering lower prices, then raised them each year by the same percentages as the high-cost indemnity plans. They were careful to stay just a little cheaper than the competition (in its shadow), thus protecting their price advantage in order to attract new business. Many employers were rudely surprised to find that the HMO that offered such a great initial rate was showing no apparent discipline in its premium increases. Honeywell calculated that such shadow pricing raised its premiums by 19 percent per year, or $10 million over a three-year period.[6]

The HMOs argued that they were fighting the same battles against costs as everyone else, but in many cases their handsome profits belied that explanation. Those HMOs did not have enough competition in their markets. As more patients signed up with such plans and larger chains began to develop, the competition grew fierce in many markets. Some HMOs cut their premiums by as much as 50 percent when Brand X moved into town. Now that more than forty-five million people are in HMOs, and some prestigious medical institutions, from Mayo to New York Hospital and Northwestern, are getting into the business, the providers are facing stiffer competition nearly everywhere, and prices are tightening up. Getting more consumers into these managed-care plans will turn up the pressure on costs across the board. At the same time, the arrival of the first-class medical institutions in managed care should improve the quality.

Ensuring the quality of care is another issue, though. Price comparisons do not tell the whole story. By practicing prepaid medicine, HMOs are able to set an annual budget and then require their staff doctors to stay within it, juggling decisions about how to care for the plan's patients and managing the costs. Nevertheless, some HMO doctors are giving better care than some higher-priced fee-for-service doctors. More medicine is not always better care. One example: HMO doctors control access to specialists and surgery. That can be seen as a limitation on quality care, but that is not necessarily true. Tens of thousands of patients die every year during unnecessary operations. The doctor who prevents an unnecessary operation may be saving the patient's life. The best-managed health plans are beginning to prove that sometimes quality actually costs less, whether the physician calling the shots is an independent fee-for-service doctor or an employee of a managed-care plan. Price does not equal quality. That should come as a relief to everyone who worries that a national reform plan will inevitably mean a decline in the quality of their medical care. It does not have to. It is possible to restrain costs while enhancing quality. It is just harder.

11

GUARANTEEING QUALITY

Everything must be made as simple as possible. But
not one bit simpler.

— ALBERT EINSTEIN

IMAGINE the ideal health-care system. We would save
money, but we would not have to cut corners or sacrifice
quality. You could go to the best doctors. You could even go
to the Mayo Clinic, and it would not cost too much.

This health system already exists. The Mayo Clinic probably provides the best hospital care in the country. It is also
the cheapest. There can be no better proof that cutting costs
does not have to mean second-rate medicine.

How is it possible? The Mayo physicians have learned
how to provide superior medicine more economically. By
relentlessly analyzing how they care for people, asking patients how the treatment turns out, and searching for ways
to improve what they do, they have learned how to do a
better job without wasting money.

Medicine is like a maze with more than one solution.
Some decisions lead to failure, but often there are several
different paths that will lead to the goal of making the patient better. Two doctors working in offices side by side may
approach someone's medical problem in very different

ways, each plan of treatment well grounded both in science and in what the doctors have learned by treating patients. In fact, studies have found that when presented with the same symptoms, ten doctors may well come up with as many as ten, or even twelve, different answers. Which one is right? Nobody knows. Each of them may solve the problem, but which way is the best?

While one physician prescribes coronary bypass surgery for a heart patient, another doctor believes that exercise and nutrition can solve the problem. Both doctors may be right; both may save the patient's life, but coronary bypass costs a lot more. In Manhattan, a psychotherapist decided early in 1993 to avoid bypass surgery. He had already had it once, and the bypass, a small piece of vein feeding fresh blood to his heart, had collapsed. His doctor wanted him to have the operation again. The patient talked to Wayne Isom, surgeon-in-chief of New York Hospital's cardiothoracic department. Isom, who has performed nearly ten thousand bypass operations, advised the patient to try exercise and a new diet. He kept a close eye on the patient's progress. In September 1993, the patient came to Dr. Isom's office to look at some new X-ray videos of his heart. "Look at that! Look at that!" said the excited surgeon. A whole new cluster of feeder arteries had developed in the patient's heart, like spring growth. Isom told his patient: "Those new arteries are providing more blood to your heart than any bypass could."

As health costs have become so burdensome, medical researchers have begun to scrutinize how doctors make decisions and how those decisions work out for patients. At the Mayo Clinic, in Rochester, Minnesota, physicians maintain that they must always answer a few basic questions when taking care of people: Is this treatment necessary? Will it make the patient feel better? Is this the best way to help the person? Finding out the answers is called outcomes research, a term for the study of how all kinds of medical treatments affect patients. Put another way, outcomes analysis is the search for the best way through the medical maze.

Until now, this type of research has been the uneasy stepchild of medicine, the blending of systems analysis and healing that no one welcomed in the operating room. Most doctors have been loath to have their judgments and results compared to those of other physicians. Who were these computer nerds who dared to challenge their life-and-death decisions? The only measures of quality that physicians embraced were as basic as mortality: did the patient survive the procedure? If the answer was yes, the treatment was successful. But even assuming that the patient lived for many more years, that left a gap in reasoning as vast as the Milky Way. What if the patient did not need the treatment in the first place? Or what if a particular treatment left the patient unable to work or to carry on normal living activities? Was there a better way?

The word "doctor" comes from the Latin "docere," which means "to teach." But doctors have resisted pooling their knowledge and teaching one another the daily lessons they learn about helping patients. Those two typical doctors working in adjacent offices usually are not even aware that they do things differently. Based on his exhaustive studies of medical practice, Paul Ellwood believes that as much as half of all medical care is of uncertain value. Even if he is right, that does not mean that none of it should have been done. Part is unnecessary, but not enough is known to be sure which part. What is certain is that medical practice varies from town to town, even from room to room.

Studies at the Rand Institute, at Dartmouth, Duke University, the Intermountain Institute for Health Care Delivery Research, and other leading quality centers have established some surprising patterns in medical practice. Dr. John Wennberg of Dartmouth documented large variations in the number of tonsillectomies, hysterectomies, and other operations performed in different areas of New England. Examining the way physicians practice medicine in Vermont, he found that while in one town 70 percent of children underwent tonsillectomies, a nearby town did them about half as often. There were no apparent reasons for the discrepancy. Comparing inpatient hospital treatment on a per capita basis, Wennberg discovered that Boston spent twice as much as New Haven did. Since the health status of the two populations is roughly the same, the question naturally arose as to whether Boston physicians were overdoing it.

Again and again, researchers have demonstrated a clear relationship between the number of surgeons in a particular place and the number of operations that are done. A medical map of the United States would show hot spots from Los Angeles to St. Louis to Chicago to Boston and New York where extraordinary numbers of procedures are performed. Kansas City has made itself the General Motors of regional coronary care, performing operations at an enormous rate. Fourteen different Kansas City hospitals offer bypasses and heart valve replacements and perform thousands of angioplasties every year, far above the per capita averages in most cities. In some parts of the Northeast, where large numbers of teaching hospitals and specialists are clustered, per capita hospitalization rates are three times as high as they are in parts of the Southwest where there are fewer major hospitals.

It seems, somehow, that whenever a specialist comes to town, the townsfolk discover that they need whatever he does. When doctors are overly eager to provide care, patients are more likely to accept it, since they have no way of judging whether it will really do them any good. In any other sort of market, supply tends to find its natural level, beyond which demand will not sustain more production.

But medicine is different. As Daniel Callahan, president of the Hastings Center in Briarcliff Manor, New York, puts it, "We have let ourselves be seduced by the idea that there is no such thing as enough health care."[1]

At the Rand Corporation in Santa Monica, Dr. Robert Brook and his associates have documented other disturbing implications of this principle. Conventional wisdom held that patients were better off choosing expert surgeons at teaching hospitals. Generally it is true that teaching hospitals do superior surgery. Doctors really are like baseball players: some are better than others. The more experienced surgeons at teaching hospitals are often more skilled at what they do. But in an extensive study of carotid endarterectomies, an operation that unclogs neck arteries in order to prevent strokes, Dr. Brook discovered that the specialists who do the most surgery also tend to do more questionable operations. As he put it, "High-volume physicians may perform a procedure better, but the patient may have been less likely to need it in the first place."[2]

There are many reasons why high-cost treatments are sometimes given to the wrong patients. Some doctors are tempted when they can resolve a murky question by performing a medical service for which they will be paid. But greed probably does little to explain the differences in the numbers of procedures that doctors perform. Professional curiosity explains some of it. In some areas of medicine, a significant amount of questionable treatment can be attributed to experimentation, as doctors try to learn by doing. The training of physicians does not end when they graduate from medical school. New therapies are constantly introduced that hold forth the promise of saving lives. Somebody has to figure out how to use them best. Doctors admit that every new test and surgical technique is overused until they learn how to do it well, and when to employ it. Physicians call this "chicken soup medicine," a reference to the old joke about how sick people should always be given chicken soup, no matter what ails them. Why? "Can't hurt."

Physicians admit, for example, that the introduction of MRI machines in the 1980s led initially to vast overuse, even more so after consumers read about them and demanded the snazzy new $1,000 test. The MRI could produce pictures of the patient's inner workings that no other test had offered and could therefore afford more precise diagnosis of many conditions. Since the scanner can make it possible to avoid invasive testing and hospitalization, a certain amount of controlled experimental excess was probably justified. The problem was that the experiment was not controlled; nearly everybody was trying it out. The same pattern has held for other diagnostic advances. In the case of prenatal tests, expectant mothers now expect to see "baby's first picture" on a sonogram, to learn the baby's sex in advance, and to be tested for detection of possible congenital defects or fetal difficulties. As a result, costly sonograms and fetal monitors are used out of all proportion to the actual incidence of evidence that they are needed. One 1993 study estimated that $1 billion in useless sonograms is being done every year, in part because patients have come to expect them, so that now doctors fear malpractice suits if they don't employ them.

In a 1988 study of coronary angiographies, a method of diagnosing blockages in heart arteries, Dr. Brook maintained that 17 percent of the procedures were inappropriate, while another 9 percent were highly questionable. Research on coronary bypass operations during the early 1980s led him to conclude that only about half did much good, though subsequent advances in the techniques have probably eliminated much of that wasteful treatment. New studies of the procedure are currently under way.

Based on his research, Brook believes that as much as 25 percent of all medical care given to insured Americans falls into a questionable area in which the likely benefit to the patient may not exceed the medical risk of complications and side effects. He says it is impossible to know yet whether his extrapolation is correct. Still, numerous studies have turned up significant patterns of dubious surgery. In a review of heart pacemaker implants performed in the Philadelphia area, Dr. Allan Greenspan concluded that 20 percent were inappropriate, while another 36 percent were debatable. This is not just a question of costs. Hospitals are dangerous places: roughly 20 percent of hospital patients go home with an infection or other problem they did not have when they went in. Worse, tens of thousands of Americans die every year during operations that probably are not necessary. Take the example of carotid endarterectomies, which are performed as protection against strokes. Of the 1,302 Medicare patients who underwent this operation in a single year, almost 10 percent died or suffered a stroke during the operation or immediately afterward. Considering that the Rand study concluded that fewer than half of the endarterectomies in its sample were clearly appropriate, while a third were plainly ill-advised, it's obvious that chicken soup medicine can kill you.

Beyond the chicken soup explanation, it is always difficult to pin down why competent surgeons perform operations or deliver other treatment that a panel of experts would challenge. Paul Ellwood argues that doctors are simply ignorant of what other physicians are doing. Robert Brook, who heads health sciences research for Rand and practices at UCLA Medical Center, has theorized that hubris plays a role in unnecessary care. He says that doctors often are excessively confident that patients can benefit from their particular expertise.

Brook also maintains, along with many other physicians, that the rapid advances in medical knowledge over the past twenty years have made it impossible for doctors to sort out all of their treatment options with complete certainty. They order tests with which they are not entirely familiar, and given a choice, may order five or six in a related series of tests because they are not sure which is precisely the right one. Besides, the insurer will pay. Sometimes compassion may play a role. Doctors want to help people. Moreover, they are supposed to know what to do. As Brook sees it: "When you go to your lawyer to discuss a complicated problem, you would not be terribly surprised if he referred to a law book while he was considering what to do. But can you imagine what people would think in the doctor's office if he took out a medical book? Doctors are supposed to have the answers; they went to medical school. But the truth is, even if the doctor pulled out the book after you left, he might not get anywhere. A lot of what we deal with every day is not in the medical books yet. It is too new." Fear contributes as well, in the form of the unnecessary care that is called defensive medicine. Doctors dread malpractice suits that can ruin their reputations and tie them up in court for years.[3]

Brook and other outcomes researchers hope to gather enough data so that they can devise reliable standards of medical practice, guidelines that all physicians can use in treating their patients. Such guidelines could help to answer the questions: when a treatment is appropriate, which treatment is best, and how it should be done. Doctors are always looking for good data. If something works consistently, they are usually willing to try it. In order to devise such broad frameworks, physicians must share information so that it can be analyzed.

No practice guidelines, of course, can replace physician judgment with textbook answers. The most difficult thing about medicine is that every human being is different. Doctors cannot know every relevant fact about a patient's condition; they can only listen to the patient and use the diagnostic tools at their command and their skills of observation to make the best judgments they can. But such practice standards could go a long way toward making some parts of medicine more routine. They could also help to eliminate defensive medicine and curb the mounting costs of malpractice insurance. At this point, personal injury lawyers are allowed, in effect, to define appropriate medical practice through massive lawsuits. If the jury agrees with the lawyer, the medical practice was wrong. Malpractice insurance premiums for doctors have tripled since 1982, rising from $1.7 billion to $5.6 billion.[4] No one is sure, though, just how much defensive medicine is practiced. The savings could run anywhere from the $20 billion that medical societies estimate, based on surveys of physicians, to several times that much, since defensive medicine has become so deeply ingrained in doctors.

Above all, outcomes researchers hope to improve the quality of medical care. In medicine, quality means providing the right diagnosis and treatment, promptly and competently. No unnecessary tests or operations, no wasteful procedures, amenities, or incompetence. No delays in giving patients what they need. And no need to operate a second time because the first procedure was not done right or was not the right one. Several states are beginning to build huge data bases on the results of medical treatment. New York now publishes annual reports on the outcomes of all bypass surgery performed in the state. Patients can look up individual surgeons to see how they have performed. Some doctors, having initially fought the idea for the reports every step of the way, now proudly display their results. The scorecards have also boosted the average quality of coronary care in the state by pinpointing mediocre surgeons. When the reports turned up heart surgeons whose operations were resulting in unusually high numbers of deaths, some hospitals withdrew the surgical privileges enjoyed by those doctors, barring them from performing bypasses. New

York will soon begin publishing data on other kinds of surgery.

One lesson from the New York research is that doctors who do complex operations relatively infrequently often do a bad job. The New York physicians whose records were poor did fewer bypass operations than those in the major teaching hospitals. Many doctors think the solution is to assign complicated surgeries to centers of excellence wherever possible. In California, 120 different hospitals perform open-heart surgery, which can include bypass operations, heart valve replacements, and other procedures. Some of the hospitals are performing fewer than two hundred of these operations every year, while others are doing well over a thousand. Mortality statistics clearly show that some of these hospitals are providing lower-quality surgery: more of their patients are dying. Alain Enthoven says: "I think the answer is that California should only allow thirty or so hospitals to perform these operations. That would be more than enough, and the result would be better quality." Even without a national reform law, some states are beginning to press for such changes.

The next step in this quality research is to involve the patients more deeply in decisions about optional surgery. Several research groups are studying when it is best to perform prostatectomy, the operation that removes all or part of the prostate gland in men. After the prostate cancer panic a couple of years ago, the rate of this surgery increased rapidly. But some doctors cautioned that too many elderly men were having the operation. Particularly in men seventy-five and older, there is not much point, if the cancer has just begun to develop. At that age, it grows very slowly and is extremely unlikely to kill them. Somewhat younger men often have the operation to correct embarrassing problems like frequent urination. But the surgery can cause unpleasant side effects, including impotence in some cases. Once patients understand what is at stake, many decide to forgo the surgery if their health will be about the same either way. In one study conducted by Dartmouth's Dr. Wennberg, men considering radical prostatectomy (the removal of the entire gland) were shown an educational video about the operation. In the video, men who had undergone the surgery explained what patients could expect, while doctors outlined the problems that might result, as well as the potential benefits of forgoing the surgery. At hospitals in Seattle and Denver, 40 percent to 50 percent of the patients decided against the operation, in part because their health would be about the same either way.[5] The video is interactive, so that the person watching the video can answer questions at certain points (such as his age and medical condition) that prompt the video to focus on information relevant to him. In this way, the patient can receive a more precise analysis of the situation he may experience. An added benefit of using interactive video: researchers can learn more about what patients want, since they can correlate the questions people ask with the final decisions they make. Doctors can use such knowledge to counsel patients. In association with Sony, Wennberg's team is preparing similar videos to help patients take part in other medical decisions. The videos will address subjects such as whether to go ahead with cataract surgery, whether to have a hysterectomy, or whether to bear a child by natural vaginal birth after previously having a cesarean section.[6]

Finally, to make sound judgments on medical quality, someone must keep track of how the patients do after they leave the hospital. In limited studies, outcomes researchers around the United States have been following patient recovery for years. One study has been under way since 1973 at the Sisters of Providence Hospital in Portland, Oregon, which has tracked patients who received artificial heart valves. Over the last several years, dozens of companies, including AT&T, Digital Equipment, GM, and GE, have tried out patient questionnaires designed by Rand's Dr. Brook and others to find out how patients suffering from such typical medical problems as lower back pain, heart disease, and asthma respond to treatment. Patients with lower back pain, for example, are asked whether they can walk up stairs easily or pick up something without difficulty. Heart patients are asked whether they need to sleep sitting up at night. The idea is to find out what sort of impact medical treatment has on the patient's quality of life. This information can also reveal where medical treatment may be falling short: should that heart patient have to sleep in his easy chair every night?[7] Eventually, the answers might also help draw the line between futile care and treatment that can make a difference. For the majority of patients, it will help sort out the differences between the treatments that are available.

These patient surveys are part of the Jackson Hole Group's approach to making health plans accountable for their quality. President Clinton, Congressman Jim Cooper, and other sponsors of reform proposals based on managed competition want input from patients to be included in report cards that would summarize information ranging from how well a health plan's doctors do to what the patients think of the outfit. The report cards might be published as community directories. Eventually, they might be made available as interactive videos. Before long, it may even be possible for Americans to find out as much about their health plan as they can already learn about the new car they are thinking of buying.

Meanwhile, the researchers are working on one piece of the puzzle at a time. In Salt Lake City, Intermountain Health Care, a chain of hospitals formerly run by the Mormon Church, has conducted a landmark study of Medicare treatment that demonstrates just how dramatically hospital efficiency and costs vary across the United States. Dr. Brent James, executive director of Intermountain's Institute for Health Care Delivery Research, says, "Our analysis shows that the cost of medicine depends very heavily on one's choice of state and hospital."

The researchers analyzed all 10.3 million hospitalizations of Medicare patients in the United States during the year that ended in September of 1991.[8] They screened out the major factors that might account for normal price differences among hospitals, including the local cost of living and the institution's investment in medical education. What was left was a clear picture of bang for the buck in medicine. Treating the same kinds of patients, hospitals in Oregon, Utah, and New York charged prices 13 percent to 19 percent below the national average, while those in Nevada, Hawaii, and New Jersey charged 16 percent to 20 percent more than average.

James and his colleagues were delighted to see that Intermountain's hospital in Salt Lake City was the second most economical in the nation. But Mayo came in number one, right at the bottom of the list. The Clinic has reported that since 1988, while U.S. per capita health spending grew by an average of 9.6 percent annually, Mayo's costs rose by only 4.8 percent per year. In 1993, Mayo's costs rose by only 3.9 percent.[9]

The Mayo Clinic spends $200 million a year on medical research and forgives the bills of patients who cannot pay; those items were factored out of hospital costs in the Medicare study. Since many desperately ill people go to the Clinic because of its reputation for diagnostic and clinical excellence, Mayo treats people who are sicker on average than other American Medicare patients and who therefore must spend more days in the hospital. The study accounted for that, too, in order to level the basis of comparison for all hospitals, big and small, simple and complex. The results show that the more rigorously good physicians work together to analyze what they do and try to learn from one another how to do it better, the more successful and cost-effective they can be.

The Mayo Clinic has been able to force down its underlying costs over many decades, through a relentless program of quality control. Mayo helped pioneer quality research in medicine. The Clinic has collated records for every one of the more than 4 million patients it has treated since 1883. Through the years, Mayo physicians have regularly combed those records, analyzing the Clinic's history of coping with particular medical problems, sometimes in patients treated over a period of half a century or more. The Clinic regularly issues papers on its findings and is now probing more deeply through computer analysis of its records, looking for other guideposts on what works best in each kind of medical situation. Since the Clinic stays in touch with its patients, it is often able to find them when new questions arise about how a particular type of treatment has worked out. This information is shared with all of the doctors at the Clinic. Every case is approached as an important research opportunity.

Perhaps the main reason that Mayo's costs are lowest, though, is that the Mayo physicians collaborate unusually closely and share an almost theological dedication to medical quality. The Clinic culture emphasizes humility, simplicity, and excellence. Physician salaries are moderate. There are no obvious signs of rank. A visitor is surprised to find that the Mayo Clinic does not look like a monument to medical ascendancy. Its hospital has changed little since it was built in 1956. The linoleum is ancient but spotless. The furniture is worn.

The thousand Mayo physicians work in simple surroundings. Their interchangeable offices are tiny and spartan.

Each is basically an examining room, with an examining table, a sink, some simple lab equipment, and a small triangular desk shoved in one corner. Anyone can drop by to consult on the patient being treated. Unlike the ranking specialists at many teaching hospitals, who enjoy luxurious, heavily paneled private dining rooms, the Mayo physicians and adminstrators eat plain food in a simple cafeteria. Says one: "I know we don't have the perks that most doctors do. But we do have one perk that no one else can match: whenever I meet someone, I can say that I am from the Mayo Clinic."

The ethic of simplicity extends to everything they do. Mayo physicians do not wear white coats. They believe in dressing like ordinary people, to remind themselves that they are, and to break down the barriers between doctors and patients. Every administrator, from the chairman on down, has a listed home telephone number, so that anyone can reach him or her at any hour. People around Rochester know them; when Dr. Robert Waller, the chairman, strolled down the street not long ago with Supreme Court justice Harry Blackmun, a former Mayo legal counsel, a woman called out, "Hey, Harry! How've you been?" The two men stopped to chat with her.

A day in the life of a Mayo physician is a constant round of patients, consultations, and meetings. They discuss everything collectively, constantly popping in to examine one another's patients and comparing notes at the end of the day, looking for ways to improve on their methods. "Nobody with a big ego lasts long around here," says Jane Campion, an administrative nurse. "Everything is teamwork. It would drive some people crazy, always having everyone else looking over their shoulder and volunteering helpful suggestions."

Not only are clinical decisions subjected to nonstop analysis, every conceivable expense is repeatedly discussed, through tiers of interlocking physician committees that closely examine the merits of the investment. A new building; a new diagnostic technique; a new high-tech machine; everything is talked into the ground, balancing probable clinical advantage against cost. Two years ago, when one doctor came up with a way of substantially improving the accuracy of a PSA, the diagnostic test for prostate cancer, the response from his fellow physicians was uncharacteristic of big-league medicine. After all, at a time when millions of men were suddenly convinced that they needed the test, thanks to the personal testimonies of cancer survivors like Senator Robert Dole and others, any hospital could make lots of money by marketing a more exacting measurement and could charge significantly more for it. Instead, the Mayo committees wanted to know what running the new test would cost. When it turned out that the added margin of accuracy was clinically meaningless and that the test would cost 10 percent more, they turned down development of the idea as wasteful.[10]

Those same thrifty budget committees approved a multimillion-dollar investment in teleconferencing equipment, so they could connect Rochester with its satellite medical centers in Scottsdale, Arizona, and Jacksonville, Florida, through two-way video. The doctors use the equipment for daily teleconsultations, peering in on patients hundreds of miles away to compare ideas. Their thriftiness never slows their focus on medical advances. During the last ten years, the Clinic has added a helicopter service to ferry patients, has established costly liver, heart, lung, and pancreas transplant programs, has built an MRI research center, and has started up a health maintenance organization. In a profession where the costs of treatment often rise in direct proportion to the concentration of specialists, Mayo does it more economically than any other American hospital with a staff that is more than 90 percent specialists and subspecialists. As it presses forward to further curb expenses and boost quality, the Clinic has a cost-saving plan that might strike some people as strange. Mayo plans to add more specialists. It works for them.

Intermountain Health Care (IHC) has taken a somewhat different approach to quality improvement, under the direction of Brent James. IHC physicians use computers to monitor and record what they do, while they're doing it. The physicians believe that if they can improve the quality of their care, patients will recover more quickly from illness and surgery. That also means that they will leave the hospital sooner and will not cost as much to treat.

One quality program has dramatically reduced one of the most common risks in all hospitals: adverse drug reactions, a term for an overdose or an allergic reaction to medicines. The Intermountain researchers discovered that in nearly half the cases of adverse drug reactions that they studied, the patient had a borderline kidney problem that the doctor had not been able to detect, one that caused the drugs to build up in the body to overdose levels. Some of the other problems were attributable to the age of the patient: older people react more strongly to drugs, so the normal dosage should be reduced. Using what he learned, James and his colleagues devised a computer program that calculates recommended dosages when a few basic facts about the patient are entered. They installed it in computers on the hospital wards. The software has been able to predict hundreds of dangerous drug problems and prevent them. Results: adverse drug reactions at the hospital have been cut in half. Since allergic reactions and overdoses can kill, the hospital has dramatically boosted quality and has saved lives.

James has also studied the way IHC physicians perform such operations as pacemaker implants, prostate surgery, and cesarean sections. He found considerable differences in the way the doctors work. He noticed that the patients treated by certain doctors ended up staying in the hospital twice as long as those treated by others for the same problems. Patients of some doctors had more complications than others did. IHC physicians explored the reasons by comparing notes and learned from the doctors with the best records of quality. James says it was not a matter of some doctors being better than others at everything. Instead, he discovered that doctors who are extremely good at one thing are often below average at something else; he tries to help them improve. He also found that some doctors who are topnotch in the morning are average in the afternoon.

One operation that he has studied is hip replacement. As a result of what Intermountain surgeons have learned from one another, their hip patients now tend to leave the hospital sooner after the operation. The average cost of the procedure has dropped by nearly 50 percent, from about $13,000 a case to $7,500.

James and his team eventually hope to study every part of the hospitalization process, including the equipment used in the hospital. When his team studied a new type of catheter approved by the Food and Drug Administration, they discovered that it wasn't all that it was cracked up to be. The catheter was supposed to reduce the number of urinary tract infections, which are common when catheters are used. One manufacturer had come up with a new catheter that was tipped with traces of silver. Silver kills bacteria. The idea was that some of the bits of silver would dissolve in the bladder, thereby preventing infections. That reasoning was good enough for the FDA, but it wasn't good enough for Intermountain.

The hospital conducted a study of roughly 4,000 patients. Intermountain doctors found that when they used the old latex catheter, 6 percent of the male patients developed infections. Using the new silver-tipped one, more than twice as many of the men (13 percent) got infections. (There was no difference for women patients.) It turned out that while the silver killed bacteria, it sometimes also irritated the bladder, causing other infections, including life-threatening kidney infections, to develop. Intermountain now plans to test every new medical gadget before allowing it to be used in its hospitals. Meanwhile, James is installing his special computers in the other twenty-three Intermountain hospitals in Utah, Wyoming, and Idaho so that the rest of his doctors can share the fruits of their colleagues' research and contribute to new studies.

In 1991 alone, the Intermountain computers in Salt Lake City saved several lives, as well as $40 million in hospital costs. But James thinks that's just the start. As he puts it: "I don't care what our quality is this year; I know it's going to be better next year, because we have worked out a successful team method for improving the way we do things. We deliver medical treatment better now, and we do it cheaper. The way things are going in health care, the only way to survive is going to be to continually examine what you are doing and figure out how to do it better."

The quality lessons that Mayo and Intermountain physicians are learning can show other American doctors how to make the critical difference between better medicine and rationing. The Mayo and Intermountain doctors have proved that doing it right the first time can save money even while improving the quality of medical care. The gains they have made in cutting their expenses have won them the opportunity to use the money they save to provide more help to patients.

Learning how to do a better job in medicine is not easy. The search for higher quality requires constant vigilance, probing self-criticism, and close cooperation among doctors. But health professionals have no choice. Rising health costs will continue to force doctors and hospitals to find ways to save money. If national health reform introduces strict spending limits for every region, it will be very difficult to make ends meet without resorting to denying patients medical care that they need. With or without national reform, the budgets are going to keep getting tighter.

The real choice in medicine today is between practicing wasteful care and efficient medicine. The difference is quality. All providers, whether small-town physicians or big-city teaching hospitals, are going to have to scramble to do the best possible job with the resources they have. Otherwise, the medical care they provide will slowly degrade, and it will become harder and harder to provide the help that patients need. At Intermountain and the Mayo Clinic, physicians believe Americans deserve better than that.

12

HOW OTHER COUNTRIES DO IT

ONE of the most common misconceptions about health reform is that easy answers are all around us, that the United
States has only to look to the wise policies of other industrialized nations to see how our health problems can be
solved. Canada is cited often. We hear that in Canada everyone gets top-quality medical care at reasonable cost. Germany is also held out as a country whose health system
works extremely well and that can teach the United States
the error of its ways. As President Clinton has noted, the
United States spends much more than these nations on
health services, yet America does not manage to cover all of
its people. He and some other U.S. leaders maintain that if
the American system were more like Canada's, or Germany's, or Britain's, we could solve our problems and also
save substantial amounts of money, enough to provide
comprehensive health care to everyone and still reduce the
national deficit.

While it is tempting to believe that we can make our way
through the anxious passage of change guided by such a
map, these assurances ignore the wrenching problems that

other countries are experiencing in trying to finance their health services and protect their quality. There are no easy answers. As the United States attempts to improve its health-care system, it can learn from the experience of other nations. The lessons include some good ideas, but also some guideposts on where things can go wrong.

Even the good ideas may not be so easy to borrow. National health policies are built not only on medical priorities, but on such social priorities as economic freedom, tax policy, personal responsibility, and acceptable limits to individual choice. These priorities define the scope of income-redistribution plans and consensus as to what matters most and what it is that citizens are willing to give up to get it. By examining the way some other nations have resolved these issues, Americans can begin to understand the choices they must consider in order to fix what's wrong with the American way of health.

CANADA'S WAY

In the 1960s, Canada nationalized its health system, creating a program called Medicare to cover all of its citizens. Medicare is a single-payer system, which means that instead of having many different insurance companies paying for medical care, the government pays the bills and finances health care by raising taxes. Because all bills go to the government for reimbursement, instead of to many different insurers, this centralized system of health care eliminates much of the paperwork. Canada's health-care system is the second most expensive in the world, after the American system.

Under the Canadian system, every citizen has health coverage and pays about 10 percent of income for the privilege.[1] People can choose their own doctors or can see specialists when they need help. The coverage includes a broad range of benefits, from preventive services like checkups and prenatal care to hospitalization, physician visits, and surgery. An estimated 63 percent of Canadian physicians are primary care doctors — focusing on family care, pediatrics, obstetrics, gynecology, or internal medicine — compared to nearly 45 percent of American doctors.[2] Everyone is promised "best care," which means that whether they are rich or poor, working or unemployed, all Canadians are promised the same level of medical services. But "best care" is not necessarily excellent care, just the best the system can afford to provide. The government regulates medicine closely, defining which services can be provided, how often, and at what cost.

Canada controls national health costs by imposing a budget and price controls on doctors and other health providers. It also tries to control costs by curbing the availability of medical services. Canada is currently reducing the number of doctors it is educating by about 10 percent as a cost-control measure. In Canada, between 1980 and 1990, taking out inflation, per capita health-care spending grew by 4.3 percent a year, almost matching the pace of spending growth in the United States.[3]

In opinion surveys, Canadians strongly endorse their medical system. Generally, they like its fairness. But Canadian doctors are deeply concerned about the growing limits on their ability to provide proper care to their patients. Canadian business leaders say the tax burden of supporting the health system is depressing employment and growth. As the federal government has shifted more and more of the financial burden to the ten provinces (health care now accounts for one-third to one-half the spending by provinces), the provinces have been forced to slash the benefits in order to slow spending growth. Several provinces now require patients to pay part of the cost of their health care as cash fees.

The Canadian system is so tightly budgeted that it often

cannot offer its citizens life-saving operations or technologies until it is too late. American cancer patients, for instance, are eight times as likely as Canadians to receive radiation therapy. Says Walter Kucharczyk, the chairman of radiology at the University of Toronto, "I can point to about a dozen cases a year at my centre where someone's health was directly jeopardized because they couldn't get an MRI."[4] Patients in Ontario wait an average of ten weeks for coronary bypass surgery; those in Quebec wait forty-nine weeks. Manitobans wait five months for cataract removal, two months for hernia repair. On any given day, 177,000 Canadians are waiting their turn for an operation or other crucial medical care.[5] Michael Walker, executive director of Vancouver's Fraser Institute, which compiled the study of waiting lists, has said: "In Newfoundland, they've solved the problem of waiting for eye operations by substituting blindness."[6]

While Canadian health care may be a little cheaper than American medicine, Canadian economists note that their country pays other costs as a result of saving on medical care, including the loss of productivity of workers who must spend more time partially disabled and waiting for help or who are never given treatment that can restore them to full health. One study, for instance, showed that because of disparities in treatment styles, Canadian heart patients were 22 percent more likely than American ones to suffer from disabling angina. Moreover, since Canadian doctors spend roughly 30 percent less time with each patient than American physicians do, they are more likely to miss signs of medical trouble. Canadian journalist Malcolm Gladwell has noted, "Because patients don't get nearly the level of attention they would receive in America, they have to come back [to the doctor] again, sixty per cent more often, taking another morning off work, wasting another hour in the waiting room, causing another round of paperwork."[7]

By contrast, the United States has too many empty hospital rooms and underused diagnostic machines. Canadian doctors say that they benefit from their proximity to the more generously proportioned U.S. health system. Canada regularly buys extra medical capacity from the United States, for instance, sending patients to Seattle or other cities for heart operations. Other Canadian patients, who can afford to pay for the privilege, simply nip over the border to such nearby cities as Detroit, Rochester, or Buffalo. As the United States considers dramatic reform of its medical system, Canadian doctors are watching with great interest. They wonder whether we will avoid the mistakes they have made. They hope we do not contract our system so sharply that they cannot continue to benefit from it. As the Fraser Institute's Michael Walker has put it: "The answer to the question, How does Canada do it? is that they do not do it. The total cost of health care is controlled by arbitrarily limiting the number of procedures of certain types, by limiting access to technology and diagnostic machinery, and by compensating physicians so that they are discouraged from responding to the demands of their patients."[8]

Ironically, even as some American political leaders are pressing to make the U.S. system more like Canada's, many Canadian leaders are urging that the only way to fix their system is to make it more like America's. The Canadian Hospital Association has called for extensive reforms of the system, with a Jackson Hole–like focus on making doctors and hospitals more competitive. Some Canadian leaders are calling for other U.S.–style changes, including the widespread introduction of HMOs.

A two-tier health-care system is growing, though many people object to the idea that some can afford things the others cannot. A fuss erupted in September 1993 when Canadians learned that more than five thousand federal bureaucrats, members of Parliament, and even government health officials use an exclusive medical clinic in Ottawa in order to obtain better service, instead of lining up with their fellow citizens for care at the local hospitals. Said one consumer critic: "Those in power don't have to wait."[9] But more and more Canadians are likely to gain access to special treatment at a price. A growing number of Canadian physicians are setting up their own privately owned diagnostic testing labs, where patients willing to pay a little more can get immediate service. The Canadian government is encouraging these developments as a way of relieving the pressure on the public system.

THE GERMAN ANSWER

Germany covers about 90 percent of its people through a system of more than twelve hundred local "sickness funds," many of which are run by private employers. (The wealthiest citizens pay for private insurance.) Germans can choose their own doctors and are covered for most preventive and emergency care, as well as funeral expenses. Employers are required to pay 50 percent of these costs for their workers. The sickness fund reimburses most of the rest of the bill. These funds are financed by 13 percent levies on worker salaries. The government pays for health care for the poorest and the unemployed. All in all, Germany devotes 8.1 percent of its gross national product to health spending.[10]

In order to limit costs, Germany imposes strict price controls on providers, closely limits the use of new technologies and drugs, and rations care to the sick and the elderly.[11] The cost pressures are growing. Reunification with East Germany means that the government must find a way to stretch resources to cover millions of new citizens. The government is now asking patients to pick up more of the cost of hospitalization and drugs. Since 1992, the government has cut back on health services. As part of the Healthcare Restructuring Act of 1993, Germany is attempting to cut costs further by forcing doctors to retire at age sixty-eight, by limiting the number of new doctors who can be licensed, curbing malpractice litigation, and capping malpractice settlements. Rationing is growing more severe.[12]

President Clinton admires the German system. So does Congressman Jim Cooper, but for a different reason. Cooper notes that German employers pay just half of the cost of health care for their workers, while President Clinton wants to require U.S. companies to pay 80 percent. Says Cooper: "The closer you get toward a hundred percent, the closer you get toward entitlement. Entitlement drives up demand and costs. In Germany, they are already having to ration care severely. We should pay attention to that."[13]

BRITISH HEALTH CARE

Since 1948, Great Britain has guaranteed basic medical care to everyone through its National Health Service and finances it through taxes. Patients pay nothing for most physician visits and hospitalizations. They pay small fees for prescriptions, eyeglasses, and dental services. Between 1980 and 1990, inflation-adjusted per capita health spending for the National Health Service rose about 2.7 percent a year, well behind the rate of growth for either the United States or Canada. Put another way, the country spends only about half as much of its gross domestic product as the United States does on health care. It shows. Long waits for doctor appointments and surgery are common, which means that some citizens cannot get lifesaving help in time to make a difference. On average, British doctors work fewer hours per week than their American counterparts do, but they see 25 percent more patients, spending markedly less time with each person.[14]

Citizens who can afford to pay more for better health care see private physicians, though they are still taxed heavily for the public system. During the last few years, concerned about declining quality and a growing need to ration medicine to make ends meet, Britain has undertaken reforms of its health system. In order to improve the quality of medicine and increase the efficiency of its health services, British officials looked to the United States for ideas. Stanford economist Alain Enthoven was among those consulted. Britain is now phasing in some American ideas about managed care, including the broad use of HMOs. The country is gradually moving toward greater privatization of health, which means that it is encouraging more of its citizens to seek care from private physicians instead of relying on the government to provide it.

SCORE ONE FOR AUSTRALIA

In the United States, where only one-sixth of students presently in medical school say they plan to become family doctors, the average young physician owes $100,000 when he or she graduates. Any idealistic yearnings to set up practice in a remote town or poor neighborhood where people need family physicians tend to fade as the young doctor considers how to pay those bills and support a family. In part for that reason, many medical students who say they plan to become family physicians change their minds by the time they graduate.

Australia has found a way to encourage more of its young medical students to choose family practice. While competition to get into medical school is rigorous, medical education is free for all citizens.[15] That means that physicians begin their careers without heavy debt and are under less financial pressure to specialize in higher-paying types of medicine. Americans could benefit greatly by emulating this idea. United States taxpayers already pay about $5 billion per year to subsidize medical schools, but only a tiny fraction of that money is providing education to family physicians. Says Dr. William Rodney, chairman of the department of family medicine at the University of Tennessee, Memphis: "I just want to get one teeny little billion of that money for American family physicians."[16]

Each of these systems offers characteristics that Americans would like to have in their medicine: universal coverage, or lower costs, or free medical education. But each of them incorporates compromises, such as rationing, that Americans may not be eager to embrace. Who makes these decisions? Physicians in other nations say that up to now, they have been able to engage in rationing without a difficult national dialogue because there was no dialogue; their citizens trust the doctors to do the right thing and do not question physician judgments as to what patients need or can rightfully expect.

Other factors also account for signficant differences between U.S. health costs and those in other nations. Canadian and German officials note that their costs are lower than America's in part because the U.S. medical system copes with different social problems. The United States pays for far higher rates of violence, teenage pregnancies (two and a half times the rate in Canada), and the tragic medical consequences of drug abuse. A Canadian study found that, considering American medicine's disproportionate social burden, U.S. health-care providers are actually doing a better job containing costs than Canadians are.[17] In addition,

11 percent of Canadians are aged sixty-five or older, compared to 12.2 percent of Americans. That may not sound
like much of a difference, but the elderly account for half or
more of almost every nation's health spending. Canadian
experts estimate that if their nation had the same proportion of older people that America does, Canada's health-
care costs would be an estimated 5.3 percent higher.[18]

Finally, because citizens in other countries do not sue
their doctors for malpractice nearly as often as Americans
do (U.S. doctors are fifty times as likely as Canadian physicians to be sued), physicians elsewhere are not forced to
engage in as much wasteful defensive medicine to protect
themselves against such lawsuits. To be sure, it is difficult to
imagine an American parent calmly accepting the notion
that a sick or disabled child cannot have a medication that
would make a difference because government officials say it
is too expensive. And what sort of lawsuit would have ensued if Stanley Roberts had been an American? In 1991,
Roberts, the former president of the Canadian Chamber of
Commerce, was admitted to Burnaby General Hospital near
Vancouver, suffering from speech problems, memory loss,
and severe headache. The symptoms indicated either a
brain tumor or an abscess. He was put on a waiting list for
tests that would identify his problem. He died before he
could get the tests. An autopsy showed that his problem had
been an abscess, which could have been cured with antibiotics.[19]

Professor Uwe Reinhardt of Princeton University is a
leading medical economist. He was born in Germany. He
says: "As a German, I prefer the idea that the government
makes sure that everyone has health care. It seems more
compassionate. But as an economist, I know that is not the
way to do it. That is not the way to control costs, or provide
good care."[20] Canadian and German officials are proud of
their health-care systems, but they readily concede that

Americans would probably not like their higher taxes, heavy regulation, and rationing.

The coming national dialogue about the best way to go about health reform will determine whether they are right about us. Other nations have made their choices. Now we must make ours.

13

ONE MAN'S STORY

MY father suffered a major stroke in February 1991. The hospital near his suburban home in northern California quickly got him stabilized. So quickly, in fact, that he was in and out before the Gulf War ended. We used to watch General Schwarzkopf together in the morning. My father could barely speak because of the partial stroke paralysis, but he would tell me stories about his experiences as part of General Omar Bradley's headquarters staff during World War II. He liked the brash Schwarzkopf. He reminded my father of General Patton. He told me about the time Patton arrived late one rainy night for a military confab with Bradley somewhere in France. Patton stormed up in a jeep at the last moment and stomped in wearing muddy boots. I'd heard the story so many times over the years that I could help him tell it.

My father had several serious medical problems complicating his condition, most prominently advanced diabetes. After several days, the hospital's director of social services came around to discuss a move to another facility for rehabilitation therapy. My father asked where he should go. His voice was faint. His eyes were huge with alarm. He was frightened because he was still so weak, and he knew nothing about rehab hospitals. The social worker presented a list of eight or ten recommended facilities in the Bay Area. She said they were the best places within a fifty-mile radius.

What she did not mention was that the first few choices on her short list were owned by the same firm that owned her hospital. Within a few days, my father was loaded into an ambulance and transferred to one of her picks. He remembers nothing about the trip: he was too sick, and the forty-five-minute ride did not help.

It was a brand-new place high on top of a hill. The physical therapy rooms were huge and filled with new equipment. The first day he was there, I watched a group of Medicare patients arrange their wheelchairs in a circle in the therapy room to play catch with a big blue ball. Most of them could not hold on to it, but they were trying. My father was unconscious most of the first two days.

The hospital was sunny and clean, a marketer's dream. The corridors were wide, the rooms large. Visiting members of my family kept exclaiming about what a nice place it was. Because he was so weak when he entered the place, my father remembers very little about it. What I remember is that it was very hard to get any information about his condition or to get any attention for his needs, but everyone was extremely cheerful. I began to think of them as the Stepford Nurses. No one there knew my father, or was very curious about him. His medical chart was seriously inaccurate, enough so that he was in danger of getting an overdose or even the wrong medication. But no matter that I mentioned it several times. No one was interested enough to fix it. I watched him like a hawk for several days. His personal physician told him, when called, that it was too far away to come and visit. In fact, my father had entered a link in the vast Medicare industry. Once he got there, his doctor no longer took care of him.

As it turned out, the place provided good rehabilitation services. He began to regain some movement in his left arm. Within a few weeks, they told my father he had progressed as far as he ever would, that he was "well," and that it was time for him to go home. At this point, he was still unable to walk, unable to sit in a chair for more than about fifteen minutes, and more than a little confused about where he was and how he got there. But he had used up his rehab budget, so he was classified as well enough to go home. My mother was beside herself, wondering how she could care for him.

Not long after he went home, and I had returned to my home in New York City, he had another serious medical crisis. It was a close call. He was in the emergency room for several hours before he was stable enough to be put into a hospital room. After a few days, the local hospital sent him to a very nice, attractive nursing home, which had a critical care unit on the second floor and carpeted rooms for permanent residents on the ground floor. My father was in the critical care unit. I returned to California for a few weeks to be with him.

After a short time, the friendly medical staff informed him that he was well enough to go home. My father was stunned. His diabetes was unstable. He was extremely weak. He had made very little progress in recovering from his stroke damage. The chief of physical therapy told him that he could not have any more sessions with the therapy staff, that he had progressed as far as he ever would. My father pointed out that he could not yet sit up in a chair. He demonstrated the fact that he could not get out of it without assistance. I watched him rocking back and forth, trying to get enough momentum to tilt forward onto his feet. The chief of therapy told him that this was as strong as he would ever be, and added that he should expect to decline steadily. That's just the way it was.

Other members of the nursing home staff began suggesting that perhaps he would like to live here permanently. All he had to do was change rooms and move into that nice section with the carpets on the floors. He was still too sick to grasp the layout of the place: where were those other rooms? He had seen them when I took him there in his wheelchair as we roamed around the facility. My father had been working very hard at his therapy and had even begun to believe that he could make a decent recovery. Now he was frightened into passivity. He said he might like to stay here rather than go home. He said it might be better for my mother. He would need a lot of help, and she did not deserve the burden. He was still under the impression that the medical staff was simply trying to help him.

I went to see the head of the nursing home, pleading with him to allow my father to stay a few more days in the medical unit. He was not stable, I said. His blood sugar was shooting up and down. He had fevers. His blood pressure was fluctuating sharply. He could barely sit in a chair without falling over. I assured the executive that my father was eager to go home as soon as possible and that he would gladly pay out of his own pocket for the cost of additional care until then. I did not know at the time that there were tight legal restrictions on what the institution could accept in private payment. Those limits were put in place by legislators who wanted to prevent hospitals from overcharging patients and defeating the purpose of Medicare price controls. The consequences have rolled through the medical system, creating an unspoken set of rules about when a patient must be released, before the hospital's losses begin to mount. This form of price controls has now redefined the meaning of the words "sick" and "well."

The nursing home administrator told me crisply that my

father had received precisely the care he needed and would be just fine leaving on schedule. He ticked off my father's medical problems on the fingers of his left hand, adding up the days allotted under Medicare for each condition, as if that would reassure me.

"You forgot Parkinson's," I said.

"Oh! Well. Five more days," he said.

He was quite pleased with himself. He had found a way to satisfy a customer. He seemed entirely unaware that he was speaking so callously, weighing my father's health like so much hamburger. What he was telling me, in effect, was that if Medicare would pay for a certain number of days, then that was the number of days it would take my father to get well. Otherwise, the nursing home would lose money. In the Medicare system, the judgment as to when a patient is medically stable is no longer in the hands of an objective physician. It has now been defined by government regulators who decide how much they are willing to pay for care, and reinforced by profit-making institutions that make money by serving the rapidly growing Medicare population but are unwilling to bend when a patient needs a little extra time. If an elderly man with several life-threatening conditions feels he is too weak to get out of his hospital bed and go home without risking his life, he obviously is not familiar with the Medicare rules. Even if he has the means to pay cash for an extra day or two, he cannot get it.

As it turned out, my father immediately began to get better, steeled by a stubborn new determination to get his strength back. He began to sneak down the back corridor to the physical therapy room. He steadied himself by shuffling slowly along the walls, determined to get there and do for himself what the staff would not. He got in trouble. The chief of physical therapy came up to his room and told him he could not use the therapy equipment. He repeated his judgment that my father did not need any more therapy,

could not make any more progress. My father insisted that
he was well enough to exercise so that he could get stronger. He said he wasn't afraid of falling. At this point, he was
so wobbly that this was a constant danger. The chief finally
relented but emphasized that no one on his staff could offer
him any assistance. Apparently, my father had used up his
quota of therapy sessions.

But that was all my father needed to hear. He kept wobbling down to the therapy room, tugging at a pulley to
strengthen his arm, shuffling between the parallel bars to
strengthen his leg. It got so when I arrived early every
morning, I checked the therapy room first. His nursing aide,
the woman assigned to help him wash and dress, secretly
encouraged him. He began using a walker when he was not
tooling around the corridors in a wheelchair visiting all of
the other patients and the workers in the kitchen. Overnight, he had become a firm convert to exercise. He did his
mouth exercises several times a day, trying to regain the
ability to speak clearly.

When I would arrive in the morning to have breakfast
with him, he would already be cleaned up and dressed in
one of his Pendleton shirts. He would be parked at his door,
waiting for me in his wheelchair, sometimes napping, until
he would see me and straighten up with a smile. "Let's go
for a spin!" he'd say. We would tour the place, visiting his
new friends, and going outside for a while to sit in the sun
and the fresh air and talk. We got to know each other for
the first time as friends. He told me about what it was like
serving in France and Germany during World War II. He
told me about his childhood. He told me about working for
his father, about the time his truck tipped over and he had
to get a team of horses to pull it out of a ditch. We talked
about how the Soviet Union was literally falling apart,
about the American economy, and business conditions. I'd
bring in some lunch and eat with him. We ate dinner to-

gether, too. He stopped worrying so much about the stroke paralysis that still made it difficult for him to eat without spilling his food. His appetite was coming back. He asked for bigger rations. After some tense discussion, the nutritionist agreed to let him have a little more food. He was regaining a few of the nearly fifty pounds he had lost during his brush with death.

The nursing staff began to call him the Mayor. He was mediating disputes between senile patients. When one elderly man with advanced Alzheimer's began hitting a woman patient who suffered from the same condition, my father interposed his wheelchair between theirs and talked the man into calming down and returning to his room. He thought it was pretty funny one afternoon when a confused woman wandered into his room, mistaking it for her own, and crawled into his bed. (He watched this from his chair.) When he was ready for a nap, he plopped into an empty bed nearby, but he told that story for days. He made friends with a retired doctor whose wife was in the final stages of Alzheimer's in a room down the hall. He tried to comfort the man, but mostly he enjoyed talking to him about what was going on in the world. They had long conversations every afternoon when the doctor visited. My father was no longer talking about wanting to stay there forever; he was now terrified that he would be forced to do so. On one of his last afternoons there, he cried, telling me that it made him very sad to spend all of his time "with all of these old people. They're sick. Nobody visits them. I want to go home."

He did, and he beat the nursing home's budget deadline, so they made a profit on him after all. He wasn't finished with medical disasters, though. He had one more major crisis the following summer. In 1992, on the Fourth of July weekend, he was transferred immediately after major abdominal surgery from a large hospital to the same sunny little nursing home.

This time, the doctor in charge of his case — who is a corporate officer of the nursing home — was away on vacation. So was the doctor who had agreed to cover his patients for him. Nobody was checking on my father. I was on the other side of the country, listening to an extremely weak father try to reassure me that he was just fine but that he couldn't talk right now. Sometimes he did not know who I was. The nursing staff objected to putting my calls through. I caught a plane for California. Before I could get there, a coincidence saved my father's life.

Our longtime family physician, the general practitioner who had cared for all of us for forty years, had died a few years earlier. His widow was a retired registered nurse. Just as my father was undergoing his latest surgery, she had a stroke. Unable to return to her home alone and needing physical therapy, she was sent to the same nursing home where my father was now slowly dying. She wheeled herself up to visit him and was astonished by his condition. His surgical incision was badly infected. She said she could smell it before she entered the room. He had pneumonia, fevers, wildly fluctuating blood sugar and blood pressure. She said the nurses wouldn't listen to her because she was a patient. By the time she managed to get a doctor's attention, my father was slipping into diabetic shock. Back he went to the hospital that had discharged him too early in order to save money. It was a week before he could leave there again. Back he went to the pretty little nursing home that had almost killed him. He was beginning to like the place. He knew everybody by their first name.

He made it. Along the way, he broke a deeply ingrained, lifelong habit of blindly trusting anyone in a white coat. I think it was even harder than back in 1974, when he had to admit that Nixon was a creep. Now he learned that not all doctors and hospitals are the same, that sometimes you're just a profit-and-loss item, and that, sometimes, just about the only person who can help you get better is yourself.

He lives in California. I live in New York. The man who by 1991 was so weak that he had taken to sleeping all of the hours except, roughly, 11 A.M. to 4 P.M., now rises every morning at 4 A.M. and makes himself breakfast. He is very quiet so he won't wake my mother. He gives me a call, talks about the news. "What do you think about this gays in the military thing?" he asked last January. And then he surprised me. When I said I didn't think it was any big deal, since gay men have been serving forever, often with high distinction, he said he agreed with me and told me about the gay men he had served with in Europe during World War II.

When the morning aerobics show comes on TV, he gets out of his wheelchair and does floor exercises. He says he can do just about everything but those sit-ups. When he and my mother visit my sister and her family in another town, he leaves the folding wheelchair in the car and makes his way up her steps with a walker and a big smile.

He got himself a souped-up wheelchair, a sports model with big, rugged tires, two speeds, and a horn. He zips up and down the steep hills in his neighborhood, traveling a couple of miles to look up old friends. He's outfitted his chair with some fancy gadgets from a San Francisco bicycle shop, including a tall orange flag and reflectors so cars can see him coming. He hasn't installed the turn signals yet; he thinks that's going a little too far. I got him a megaphone in case he ever needed to call for help along the suburban sidewalks he roams. He delights in scaring the daylights out of his neighbors by using it to greet them as they drive by.

When he needs a haircut, he shoots down to a local shopping center. The women in the barber shop move one of their chairs so that he can back his chair into position for a

trim. Sometimes, he stops at the grocery store and buys my
mother a surprise, like a leg of lamb, and carries it back up
the hill to her on his lap. He weeds the garden, positioning
his chair so he can do it with his good hand. He waters the
flowers. And he always makes sure that the spare battery
for his chair is recharging in the family room so that he'll
have his wheels. The last time a doctor wanted to do a little
surgery, he said "I don't want to. Every time I start to get
better, something like this comes along and knocks me flat
for six more months. I'll take my chances." This summer,
he'll be eighty.

My father is not one of those underserved, uninsured
Americans that President Clinton is properly concerned
about. He lives in the Bay Area, which enjoys one of the
best concentrations of medical skill and facilities in the
United States. He has Medicare. He has money. His problem
was not that he could not afford coverage or did not live
near good doctors. His problem was that he needed to get
his medical help from the Medicare system.

When President Clinton was making his eloquent address to a joint session of Congress last September, outlining
the need for health-care reform, he talked about the wasteful medical bureaucracies that generate unbelievable
amounts of paperwork. Ironically, he seemed unaware that
he could well have been describing the horrors of dealing
with the huge Medicare bureaucracy. My father com-
mented the next day that he was not sure it was a good idea
to set up a far larger one for all Americans.

We've come a long way from the old days of the family
doctor. Now we have a well-meaning federal bureaucracy
that has written 300,000 pages of Medicare and Medicaid
rules on how to deliver medical help to Americans. Problem
is, those rules have nothing to do with one sick person
whose ability to recover does not conform closely enough to

the dense thickets of regulations written by government employees somewhere in Washington, D.C. And because of the complexity and price restrictions in those rules, they have discouraged family doctors from treating their patients once they enter the Medicare world.

Medicare offers an instructive model for the coming national reforms. The program was going to provide medical care for all elderly Americans. Nobody said anything about rationing. The promises have not really been kept, and the price is far higher than estimated. People are not dying as early as everyone expected. Medicine keeps on improving its methods. The population of older Americans continues to grow. The rationing is getting worse.

President Clinton has included coverage for prescription drugs for Medicare beneficiaries in his legislation, and that will come as a relief to people like my father who spend substantial amounts every month for multiple medications. The president said that it was not right for the elderly to be forced to choose between pills and food. But his legislation also requires substantial cuts in Medicare spending over the coming years, even as the population of the elderly is growing. One hopes that they will not be forced to choose between pills and doctors.

One of my most talented and prolific colleagues at *Time* magazine had a kidney transplant a few years ago. He is in his early sixties. He's still writing elegant news stories, some of them about the president's plans for health reform. We think we need him. We think he was worth saving. Would he have been saved, though, if he needed that operation in the year 1998 instead? As we engage in what President Clinton has called "the great national dialogue" about health reform, it is up to all of us to be sure he would.

14

ALL THE KING'S HORSES

Command economics didn't work in Russia, and it
won't work here.
— RICHARD SCOTT, CEO, Columbia/HCA
Healthcare

THE coming legislative battle over health care promises to
be fierce. President Clinton has staked his reputation — and
possibly his chances for reelection in 1996 — on signing a
reform bill into law. By driving hard to pass the bill in 1994,
he has also made it the bellwether issue for the candidates
running for all 435 seats in Congress and 34 places in the
Senate. Health-care reform may well be the most important
and complex legislative issue in a generation. It affects every
American personally. It would restructure a $1 trillion sec-
tion of the economy and directly affect the jobs and incomes
of fifteen million American health workers. It will affect
medical research and patient care. For better or worse, it
could redefine the American way of health.

President Clinton knew he had a tough fight ahead of
him. Throughout 1993 and early 1994, White House officials probed the arguments of those in a strong position to
support or hinder the president's proposal. No reform
would be possible unless the administration could build a

strong enough base of support while keeping potential opponents off balance. Before presenting the president's plan to Congress, the administration had added benefits that would bring key supporters aboard and softened some requirements that might alienate powerful groups. Big Labor won tax protection for its benefits, which are generally more lavish than those the White House wants to guarantee everyone else. Physicians were assured that most doctors would still be able to see their regular patients if the patients were willing to pay a little more for the choice. The American Association of Retired Persons was relieved to see that the proposal would include new Medicare coverage for prescription drugs and also would not harm its money-making pharmaceutical and insurance-selling arms. But it was those who want the United States to create a federally run, tax-funded system like Canada's who scored the biggest victory, nudging the Clinton proposal deep into regulatory territory. Health experts who had applauded President Clinton's endorsement of a market-based approach to reform were taken by surprise when they saw how his ideas had changed. They did not like his shift toward a government-controlled medical system. Stephen Wiggins, the chairman of a Connecticut HMO called Oxford Health Plans that serves 200,000 people, conceded that the White House plan could help him financially, since it would encourage everyone to join HMOs. But he still opposed the proposal, saying, "The single-payer people turned this so-called managed-competition plan into a Trojan horse. This will hurt our health system."[1]

The proposal that President Clinton presented to Congress in late October 1993 was the result of the careful, behind-the-scenes winnowing process: a blend of ideas and political compromises. By the time it was submitted a few weeks later as a House bill, another flurry of changes had been made as more compromises were struck. And still the horse-trading continues, so that it seems clear that the proposal the president delivered to Capitol Hill that October afternoon will be very different from any bill that may become law. The administration tried to conclude much of the process of compromise before the legislation went to Capitol Hill, to anticipate and account for all major objections before going public with its plan. But most potential opponents rejected that approach. They discussed their concerns with the White House, but they said that they had little confidence that agreements reached in 1993 would still be in place by the time Congress took up the legislation. A lobbyist for the American Medical Association bluntly expressed his own harsh view of the process: "Bill Clinton has no bottom line. He will sell anything for a vote. Anything the White House agrees to now may change further down the line. The real decisions will happen at the end of the legislative process. That is the final round. That is when you want to have your powder dry. And that is where we will focus our efforts." Others shared that view of how health reform will proceed, the battle growing ever more intense as the House and Senate try to agree on a final bill.

As he wages this political struggle, President Clinton has already accomplished a remarkable thing. Through his uncompromising commitment to reform, he has managed to make health care the top domestic issue and to keep it at the top of the national agenda for more than a year. He has made it politically impossible to say it cannot be done, has forced all sides to come to the table to shape a plan. Right now, despite their disagreements, the power players in politics, in business, and in medicine are still willing to march down the road to reform under the president's banner. But that will change if the political pressure for reform eases. Says Dr. Roy Schwarz, the AMA's senior vice president for medical education and science: "They will go down that road as long as the king's army is at the gate. But as soon as that army withdraws, they will go back to doing whatever they think is best."[2]

President Clinton has said that his bottom line is affordable health coverage for everyone. That is an admirable and desirable goal, but it is not an easy thing to accomplish. Like all of the major proposals for reform, the Clinton plan would require fundamental changes in the way people get their medical care, in the way they buy their insurance, and in the way that doctors and hospitals work. But the Clinton plan goes farther than most of the congressional proposals. Its central requirement is that all Americans give up some control over their private medical arrangements so that everyone can be guaranteed comprehensive coverage. Economists say the president's proposal would be expensive. The Clinton plan attempts to find the money for these changes by cutting some federal spending and by raising some taxes. That strategy will be fiercely debated.

Critics say the plan's main weaknesses are its price controls, which they say could force doctors to ration medical care and could also devastate pharmaceutical research; its requirement that employers pay most of the cost of care, which even the White House concedes will cost hundreds of thousands of jobs; and the sweeping nature of its guarantees, which they say would drive up health-care spending.

Here are the key arguments:

1. *Price controls would hurt medical quality and might cause rationing of health services*

The White House plan would impose price controls on doctors, hospitals, insurance plans, and pharmaceutical companies. Hospitals say they would not have enough money to provide medical care to everyone who would need it. Insurance companies say that the plan would prevent them from raising enough money to pay the medical bills. Doctors say the government does not have the right to force them to work for lower wages and that the plan would not give them enough resources to take proper care of their patients. Pharmaceutical companies say the price controls would prevent them from developing the new drugs they have in the works that could control some of the most devastating — and expensive — diseases.

Dr. Richard Weinshilboum, vice chair of the Mayo Clinic's board of trustees, calls the Clinton price controls "the economics of ignorance." Just when the pharmaceutical and biotech companies appear to be on track toward finding medications to control Alzheimer's disease and other devastating conditions, he argues, the federal government is putting forward a plan that hurts their chances of producing those medicines. The drug companies have already said they are going to cancel some research projects because their investors have pulled out.[3]

Senator Daniel Patrick Moynihan, the chairman of the Senate Finance Committee, which must approve the financing of the new benefits, has said that the president's provisions for paying for health care are unrealistic. If that is true, then Congress would be forced to come up with more money as health plans run out of funds. Alain Enthoven and other health experts agree. They say that by putting tight limits — caps — on the insurance premiums that pay for medical care, the Clinton plan would cause huge tax increases when Congress comes to the rescue. They insist that the best thing to do is to rewrite the entire bill and come up with a more practical approach. Otherwise, Enthoven says, "The Clinton price controls will lead fairly quickly to rationing."

"Look," says Kirk Johnson, the general counsel for the

American Medical Association. "Premium caps mean rationing. Everybody knows that. You cannot increase access to care and contain costs this quickly without cutting services to people. The president is right to attack waste and inefficiency in the health system. He knows we spend too much on futile care, but he doesn't talk about that. The problem is that instead of addressing some of those areas, he is trying to force everyone to slash their costs overnight. If you put these health plans in a real financial bind, they will crack down hard on the doctors to reduce care. That's not quality care: that's second-rate health care."[4]

Bill Gradison, the president of the Health Insurance Association of America, says that the price controls on insurance premiums are so tight that they could bankrupt regional health plans and thus endanger medical services for entire areas because they would legally prevent insurance companies from charging enough to pay the medical bills, no matter what the local residents wanted. "One of the real ironies of this approach," says Gradison, "is that to make the president's health plan succeed, we need a financially viable private sector of health providers, everybody from insurers to HMOs to group practices. Someone will have to manage the money to pay for all this health care. But in the Clinton plan, we are not being given the opportunity or the time to produce the money and the added efficiencies that will be needed to run this system."[5]

2. *The plan would cost jobs*
Critics say that because the plan requires businesses to pick up most of the cost of broad health benefits for their workers, it will force employers to eliminate hundreds of thousands of jobs. The White House has conceded that 600,000 jobs may be lost in the short run, and economists

outside the administration have projected up to 2 million layoffs. Many small companies say the new costs may drive them out of business.

Larger employers say the White House requirement that companies must provide the full complement of benefits to part-time workers means that companies will have an incentive to replace the part-timers with temps. Under the plan, they are not responsible for temporary workers' benefits. Mitchell Fromstein, the chairman of the Manpower temporary agency, the largest private U.S. employer, supports the Clinton plan. He says that it would bring him a lot of new business. Under the Clinton proposal, the federal government would pay part of the cost of benefits for part-time workers on a sliding scale according to how many hours they work. Companies say this would encourage them to replace full-time workers with part-time workers, so that the government would pay for more of the benefits. They also say they would reduce the hours that part-time employees work, because then the government would also pay more.

Since everyone in the Clinton health alliances pays the same insurance premium, people in big cities would pay higher insurance rates to cover the health needs of the inner-city poor. In order to cut federal spending on Medicaid, the Clinton plan would also require urban residents to pick up billions of dollars in Medicaid costs through their personal insurance premiums. Companies say it would be in their interest to cut back jobs in the cities so that they would not have to pay their share of those higher costs for urban workers.

3. *Many Americans will have less choice*
The president's proposal would give Americans who have little or no insurance better coverage and more choices. It would also give many other workers more options on the kind of health plan they want than they now enjoy at

their companies. But it also gives the new local health officials extensive power to limit people's choices of the doctors and hospitals that they use. That would mean these officials could refuse to cover people who wanted to go to medical centers in other states that are more expert in treating their medical problems. Some state officials say they might want to do just that, since then the medical centers in their own states could benefit by treating more people. Such planning would hurt the major medical centers in cities like Boston, New York, Atlanta, St. Louis, and Chicago, which serve many patients from nearby states. It could also hurt the Mayo Clinic, which serves patients from all fifty states.

"If we are not careful," says Dr. Robert Waller, Mayo's chief executive, "health reform could be very destructive. What I worry about most is the question of free choice and access. People come here from all over. I want to be sure that people in need can still come to the Mayo Clinic. I am not sure that will be true under the president's plan."[6]

4. *The plan will make health costs rise*

Economists say the plan would drive up overall U.S. health costs because it would insulate Americans even more than before from the real costs of medical care by placing the main responsibility for providing health coverage on taxpayers and employers. Alain Enthoven maintains: "When we put together the managed-competition model for reform, we were thinking in terms of empowerment, of making it possible for all Americans to have affordable coverage and decent health care. But that is profoundly different from the federal government reaching down from the top and telling everyone what they have to do and how they have to do it. The heart of the Clinton plan is entitlement. And entitlement always means that people want more because it is guaranteed by the government."[7]

Until now, employers have worked the hardest to control health costs, since they had to come up with the money for the employee benefits they offered. But critics say that even as the Clinton plan requires companies to pay for new benefits, it removes their incentives to find ways to control the costs. The reason: their contribution toward the cost of employee benefits will be capped, at 7.9 percent for large companies in the president's proposal. The new requirement will act like a tax. Almost no one thinks the 7.9 percent levy will cover the whole cost of benefits. (The government will pay the rest.) Therefore, employers will see no way they can save money by attacking health-care costs; they will still have to pay the same thing, even if prices go up. In Enthoven's view, "It will wipe the large employers right off the battlefield of cost control. They will say, 'OK, we'll just pay our 7.9 percent of payroll and forget about trying to fight health-care costs. That's not our problem anymore.' If you take away a company's serious and lively interest in finding ways to cut costs, you drive up costs. This plan will do that. And Congress is bound to raise the 7.9 percent payroll limit when that happens."[8]

5. *The plan contains too many hidden taxes*
Big Labor gets to keep its more generous benefits, and the Clinton plan asks everyone else to subsidize them through taxes. Congressman Jim Cooper believes: "That's great for companies like Chrysler! It's a windfall, a huge subsidy. Taxpayers and smaller firms will be forced to pay their bills. This will hurt small employers. Their workers will get less, but they will have to pay for the union benefits at the big companies."

Corporations with five thousand or more workers can choose to run their own health alliances for their employees and pay 80 percent of the costs, up to that 7.9

percent payroll limit. But if they do, they will also have to pay another 1 percent payroll tax to help support the public health plans in their area. In other words, this new tax would require companies to help pay for the health costs of people who don't work for them, as well as the salaries of the people who run the public alliances.

Younger people will pay higher insurance premiums to cover the greater health needs of the Baby Boomers and the elderly. That may be a good idea, but it will mean that younger workers are effectively taxed for the benefits of the far larger group of older people.

The federal government will save money on Medicare by forcing people in the local health alliances to pay some of the bills. The president's plan states that any Medicare beneficiary who has a job, or whose spouse does, will now receive family health-care coverage from the employer involved instead of from Medicare. If that company is part of a public alliance, all of the members of the alliance will share the new costs formerly covered by the federal Medicare program. If the company runs its own health alliance, the employer will inherit this Medicare burden. At the same time, the local alliances would be asked to pay for some ailing people who had been covered by Medicaid.

In these ways, the federal government would save money by forcing people in local areas to pick up billions of dollars of its financial responsibilities. Governor Howard Dean of Vermont, a physician, said his fellow governors are alarmed: "Why is it that every time the federal government puts its thumb on something, it ends up turning the wrong color for us? Every time the federal government gets involved in rule-making, it is inept! We don't want one big Medicare program. I believe that this president's vision of a federal health program would destroy the quality of our healthcare."[9]

6. *Malpractice litigation would increase*
   The Clinton plan guarantees everyone the right to comprehensive health care. It also gives them the right to sue doctors, health plans, and government officials if they feel they have not gotten what they are entitled to. By doing so, critics say that the plan will encourage people to sue when the health plans have trouble finding enough money to give patients everything they want, whether or not their doctors think they need it.

   Says Kirk Johnson, the general counsel for the American Medical Association: "Under this plan, you tell everyone that they have the right to the best in medical care. But the health plans that are providing health care are going to be hammering on doctors to provide less care. You're going to have patients wondering, 'Did I get everything I was entitled to?' And then they may begin to think: 'I don't feel as good as I should. I didn't get cured. Maybe they're so worried about these price caps that they're not giving me everything I deserve. So damn it, I'm going to sue!' The conflict between this concept of a universal right to best care and the premium caps, which will force rationing and make it impossible to provide the best care, will lead to more litigation. It's not honest to say we can get these benefits without talking about placing limits on medical care. It will be unpleasant to talk about that. But we need to have that public debate. It is no service to the American people to avoid it."

7. *The plan will increase waste by creating large new bureaucracies to run health care*
   The White House proposal depends heavily on cutting waste in health spending in order to come up with the money to pay for the new health-care system. The administration maintains that its plan will simplify paper-

work and reduce the bureaucracy in medicine. But congressional critics call the proposal "trickle-down health care," pointing to the amount of money it will take to support the costly new layers of state and federal bureaucracy.

Congressman Jim Cooper says: "The health system described in the Clinton plan is ruled by bureaucrats. The overreaching in the president's plan is due to the fact that our most liberal friends just can't leave well enough alone. They want the government involved in every nook and cranny of our lives." Oxford Health's Stephen Wiggins agrees. He says: "This plan represents a total lack of trust in free markets. President Clinton seems to harbor a breathtaking blind faith that the government can and should run one-seventh of the U.S. economy."

"You don't want politicians deciding those things," says Alain Enthoven. "Vice president Gore said something relevant to this in his report on reinventing government. I've got it right here. It says: 'Public confidence in the federal government has never been lower. The average American believes that we waste 48 cents of every tax dollar.'

"Well, they're right. I believe that the federal government wastes 48 cents of every tax dollar. I don't want a system where we turn over all of our insurance money to politicians. Maybe the president should read this report."

And so the battle is joined. All sides seem to agree that 1994 is the critical year for health-reform legislation. After that, it will be hard to get everyone to agree on a plan. For one thing, preliminary scrimmaging for the 1996 presidential campaign is already beginning. By the end of 1994, political interests may begin to diverge in too many directions for sure-handed control of such a high-stakes legislative process. It may well be that the only way the president can get a bill completed is to make major compromises on such issues as the employer mandates and price controls before the moment passes.

Sometimes it seems that all of the doctors are involved in the political debate over reform. Many people have been startled during visits to their own physicians lately, when the doctors wanted to talk about the president's plan and tell them what was best. People don't necessarily want to talk about politics with their doctors, especially when their doctors talk about money or tell them that health reform might take away medical care that patients need. "Are they worried that they're going to make less money or something?" asks one patient. "I just didn't feel comfortable. Besides, he knew a lot more about it than I did."

Some doctors are worried that a new law might reduce their incomes. But a lot of other physicians are enormously worried that once Congress starts fighting over how to change the American way of health, there is no telling what they will come up with or whether it will work at all. "What really worries me," says Paul Ellwood, "is that by the time they are finished, they may come up with some sort of unworkable perversion of all of these ideas. That would be terrible. Reform is so important, but we must be very careful not to ruin the good things about our medical system."

Brent James, at Intermountain Health Care in Salt Lake City, says he loves the practice of medicine. He has devoted his life to studying how his fellow physicians take care of patients and helping them learn how to do it better. He believes in reform. He also believes that American medicine is on the cusp of change so vast that it will rival the dawning of the space age as medical researchers drive closer to the hidden heart of disease, learning how to fix genes before they can create physical tragedy. He believes that he will see these things in his lifetime, that he will be able to bring these things to his patients.

He says: "We stand at a crossroads. We can redefine medicine and turn American health care into something the world hasn't even imagined in terms of how good it can be. We can redefine what it means to serve and what it means to be a nurse or a physician. We can achieve a level of care that has never been seen before. But if we mess it up, we can destroy this whole system. We can damage people's lives. We can increase the costs, increase the cynicism, increase the name-calling and the shouting. We can make medicine the sort of thing that people will run away from. And we are at that point of decision. What we're talking about here is the profession of medicine."[10]

It is up to all of us.

GLOSSARY

The Meaning of it All

IT is not by accident that health-care terminology is so hard to understand. That's the whole idea.

Language can obscure or clarify meaning, depending upon the intentions of those who use it. Thus medical terminology is clear, if also cold and scientific. It always means the same thing. A vein is always a vein. Not so in the language of health care, where ordinary words sometimes take on surprising meanings, and new terms may not describe what they seem to mean. The field of health care embodies more than medicine, encompassing the priorities and delivery of health services. Because there is so much disagreement about the best way to provide medicine, and so much money at stake, the language of health care is distorted by conflicting sales pitches.

Caught between politics and business, this new language reflects the efforts of all sides to gloss over unpleasant realities and convince their audiences that their concepts are superior. Medical terms are put at the service of persuasion. While health marketers seek to spin advertising concepts like New! and Improved! into their language, politicians choose equally deceptive terms that incorporate policy visions of the way things ought to be. To an objective patient or doctor, the phrase "quality care" may mean good medicine. When the same words are used by government health officials, though, they take on a political meaning, usually indicating a medical system that guarantees to provide everyone with precisely the same services: quality means entitlement. Meanwhile, when health marketers talk about quality, they may mean consumer appeal (convenience and price, attractive surroundings, free parking). The term "health care" itself incorporates a political assumption. Substituted for "medical care," this new term embodies an assumption that physicians are responsible for keeping people healthy, however that condition is defined.

Thus the language of health care is often Orwellian. George Orwell said that political language "is designed to make lies sound truthful and murder respectable, and to give an appearance of solidity to pure wind."[1] He would find much to comment upon in the present debate over health reform.

The following glossary of health-care terms will help readers understand the language being used in the national debate over health reform.

Accelerated Benefits: An arrangement under which a life insurance company allows dying patients to cash out their benefits during the final year of life. Pioneered by the Prudential as a compassionate alternative for people with AIDS and other expensive terminal diseases.

Access: Can you find a doctor when you need one? If so, you have access to medical care. Access is not coverage.

Accountability: The notion that doctors, hospitals, and health plans should demonstrate the value of their medical services. By keeping track of how the patients feel and how the treatments affect their lives, providers would be accountable to potential customers for the quality of their work.

Accountable Health Plan: Under the Jackson Hole model of managed competition, health plans would be held accountable for the quality of their medical care so that consumers or their alliances could choose providers based on how well they perform. See **Report Card**.

Actuary: A professional expert in standard health statistics who assists in determining insurance premium rates. One survey said that actuaries have the lowest mortality rates of any profession, perhaps because their work is so predictable.

Administrative Costs: The cost of filling out insurance forms, plus all the other expenses generated by the bureaucracy of health systems, from the handsome salary of the hospital president to the pay of the legions of clerks processing paperwork on a floor somewhere below.

Administrative Simplification: The idea of simplifying the amount and complexity of the paperwork associated with medical care by eliminating some of the forms.

Adverse Selection: The phenomenon that occurs when the nature of an insurance policy or health plan attracts sicker people, on average, making it harder to spread out the financial risk of coverage. Typically seen when a plan offering generous benefits competes with a tightly managed HMO. Healthier people, who need less medical care, tend to congregate in the lower-cost HMO plan. Those who need more frequent and costly care choose the more generous plan. Adverse selection unbalances the finances of a health plan, producing levels of demand that it cannot afford to cover and driving up premiums.

Aftercare: Essentially means Somewhere-Else Care. Health services for patients after they are released from hospitals. Usually tailored to weaning the patient from treatment, aftercare deals with the problems of people who might have benefited from a couple more days in the hospital if their insurance had covered it.

Alliance: An entity that buys health services for consumers who live in its territory.

Alliance Eligible: A person who is eligible under the Clinton plan to be represented by a particular alliance. Generally, eligibility is determined by place of residence.

Allied Health Workers: Not doctors, nurses, or dentists. These specially trained workers do everything from paramedical rescue to many of the tasks formerly performed by nurses, such as drawing blood samples, taking temperatures, and giving patients medicine.

Allowable Costs: What the insurer is willing to pay for.

Alternative Dispute Resolution System (ADR): Not clearly defined, this part of the Clinton legislation is intended to resolve some legal claims against the health plans or alliances without using the courts. See **Arbitration**.

Alternative Medicine: Not covered under the Clinton plan, these are nontraditional remedies, from acupuncture, homeopathy, and biofeedback to herbal therapy. So many people swear by these treatments that Congress established the Office of Alternative Medicine at the National Institutes of Health in 1992 to study the field and try to distinguish the quality from the quacks.

Ambulatory Care: Portable patients. Medical treatment that does not require hospitalization.

American Bar Association Full Employment Act: How doctors describe President Clinton's approach to malpractice reform. They feel that his changes will only result in a storm of new litigation against doctors and hospitals. See **Enterprise Liability**.

Appropriate Care: Medical care that can be expected to help the patient. See **Inappropriate Care**.

Arbitration: A method of settling legal claims before a

court-appointed arbitrator, this procedure eliminates the need to take malpractice claims before a judge and jury. Proponents stress its cost-effectiveness. But studies suggest that malpractice awards handed down by arbitrators may be just as high as those resulting from the jury system.

Basic Care: Definition unknown. A term that purports to describe the medical care a person needs, as opposed to what he or she might like to have.

Bean Counter: Slang for those people with green eyeshades who challenge your doctor's decisions on the care you need and try to make sure the health plan does not spend too much taking care of you. See **Gate Keeper**.

Beds: Hospital beds. Hospitals calculate their capacity and costs according to how many beds they offer and the average number occupied by patients on any given day. Since a hospital with many empty beds is usually losing money, these institutions try to design their services and plan their treatment in a way that fills the beds. Insurers, meanwhile, try to avoid the costs of housing patients in hospitals. Neither side is necessarily acting in the best interests of the patients.

Biotechnology: The medical field in which scientists alter the genetic structure of plants or animals to produce desirable characteristics. By altering vegetables, biotech can make them resistant to bad weather. By altering bacteria, researchers can turn the bacteria into tiny manufacturing units making insulin or other vital medications. Biotech firms are expected to invent dramatic new remedies for disease.

Board Certified: Signifying that a physician practicing in a certain specialty has passed the boards, or final exams, of the appropriate medical society.

Bonus Sharing: A specialist working for a managed-care health plan like an HMO earns a bonus at the end of the

year if certain costs of treating patients are lower than
was budgeted.

Broken Loop: A concern expressed by family physicians.
Normally, a family doctor refers patients to specialists for
particular problems, then resumes general care as the patients return. But under a medical system that increasingly is focused on compensating doctors for primary
care, the specialists try to keep the patients referred to
them, offering to act as their personal physicians. The referral loop is broken. The family physicians are displaced
by the specialists, who present themselves as primary
physicians, even though they don't know as much as the
family doctor about many things.

Bundling: An accounting procedure by which related
medical services are reported to insurers as a single treatment, rather than being billed separately. Bundling is un-
popular with most doctors and hospitals because it
usually results in lower reimbursement. If medical treatment were a car, a bundled treatment would be billed as
the purchase of a car, rather than as the separate pur-
chases of four wheels, a carburetor, a driveshaft, some
spark plugs, and all of its other parts. See **Unbundling**.

Capitation: A set amount allotted by a health plan or insurance plan to cover a particular person's medical care
during a year.

Caps: Absolute limits on costs. An example is the premium
cap favored by the White House, which would regulate
the rate by which insurance premiums could rise and
would therefore limit the amount of money available for
health care.

Catastrophic Care: The medical care needed when a patient suffers a major injury or life-threatening illness that
requires expensive long-term treatment.

Cherry-Picking: A profit-enhancing practice followed by
some insurance companies and health maintenance or-

ganizations that try to select healthy customers whose medical needs are less expensive to cover, while avoiding covering poorer and sicker people. Small insurance companies cherry-pick by selling insurance to healthy groups and refusing to write coverage for the so-called bad risks. Since richer people are usually healthier, health maintenance organizations cherry-pick by advertising in high-income areas or by locating their offices in areas where people with good jobs and better incomes live and work.

Chicken Soup Medicine: Treatments of questionable merit. A reference to the old saying that sick people should always be given chicken soup. Why? "Can't hurt." Trouble is, unnecessary treatment *can* hurt. Every year, tens of thousands of Americans die during operations they did not need.

Child: According to the Clinton plan a child is either a son or daughter or "an unmarried dependent eligible individual regardless of age who is incapable of self-support because of mental or physical disability which existed before age twenty-one" (a disabled dependent, in other words).

Choice: Constantly promised in the health debate but limited in the Clinton plan. See **Single-Payer System**.

Closed Network, Closed Access, or Closed Panel: A health plan that dictates which doctors and hospitals can serve its members, usually as a cost-control measure.

Code Creep: The subtle tendency of doctors and hospitals to describe the medical services they provide in insurance codes that yield maximum reimbursement. Code creep happens when a common procedure, perhaps a physician's office visit, begins to be reported consistently as an extended visit. See **Upcoding**.

Coding: An accounting procedure by which medical services are described in insurance codes (numerical names), to identify them for the designated insurance reimbursement. An ordinary doctor visit, for example, has a certain code, while an extended visit, during which the physician takes more time to explore troubling signs, has a different code and pays more.

Coinsurance, Copayment: Your share. The portion of medical costs that the patient must pay. This awkward term came into common usage as companies and insurers began to shift more of the costs of medical care to patients. Copayments are the small fees that the patient must pay when visiting the doctor or picking up a prescription.

Commercial Insurance: Insurance offered by profit-making firms. These are companies like MetLife, Aetna, and the Prudential that try to generate profits for their shareholders.

Community Rating: Everyone has the same insurance rates. Required under the Clinton and Cooper plans, this is a method of setting insurance premiums that reflect the health needs of everyone in a given area, rather than varying the prices according to the age and health of individual beneficiaries. Hawaii already requires community rating. Proponents like it because it eliminates extreme variations in premiums and spreads the burden of medical costs over a larger population. Opponents object because younger, healthier people must pay higher rates to cover the costs of caring for older or sicker people.

Comprehensive Care: A vague term for coverage of virtually everything from preventive care to hospitalization. Like many health euphemisms, this one is open to wide interpretation and implies misleadingly that all benefits will be included. Among the many things excluded from the comprehensive care in the Clinton proposal, for instance, are glasses and dental checkups for adults.

Congenital Anomaly: An acceptable excuse for cosmetic

surgery, as defined by the Clinton plan. Of course, everyone sports congenital anomalies, which are odd personal characteristics that were inherited. Who will decide which ones are important enough to merit coverage of surgery to correct them? It will be up to government bureaucrats and lawyers to sort this one out.

Conversion: The right to change one's insurance coverage from participation in a group policy to individual coverage without having to take a new medical examination to qualify for the insurance.

Cookbook Medicine: Doctors who do not want to cooperate with quality research say the result would only be stupid rules telling physicians how to take care of patients. They deride such rules as "cookbook medicine." See **Practice Standards**.

Coordination of Benefits: When a husband and wife have separate insurance coverage, usually through their employers, questions arise as to which insurer is responsible when someone in the family seeks medical treatment. In coordinating benefits, the insurers determine which policy bears the principal burden of coverage. This practice, which most insurers dislike as time-consuming, is intended in part to prevent people from unethically duplicating claims, sending the same bills to both insurance companies and making a profit.

Core Benefits: The benefits that everyone gets under a health plan, as opposed to additional benefits that an individual or company may pay more to get.

Corporate Alliance: A health-care purchasing alliance run by a corporation to serve its own employees.

Cost-Shifting: A way of making up losses in one area by charging more in other areas. Often used to describe what happens when people without insurance go to the emergency room. The hospital makes up the expense of treating them by padding the bills of those who have insurance, usually by charging higher prices. See **Playing Robin Hood**.

Coverage: Insurance. A guarantee to pay a certain share of the cost of specified medical services. Not to be confused with care. See **Access**.

Creative Accounting: Padding the bill. Some doctors and nurses attend special seminars to learn how to express the medical services they render in the most expensive possible terms on insurance forms. Consultants specialize in showing them how. See **Upcoding, Unbundling**.

Cross-Subsidizing: Covering some costs by raising prices on others. Hospitals, for example, traditionally have covered their losses on Medicare and Medicaid treatment and bolstered their funding for research and training by charging people with good insurance more. Managed care tends to eliminate cross-subsidization by watching all costs more closely. As a result, many hospitals are hard-pressed to find the money for things like training and treatment of the uninsured.

Custodial Care: Generally a reference to nonmedical services provided by nursing homes or home health aides to people who require assistance in ordinary daily activities such as dressing and cooking.

Day Surgery: A term for operations that can be performed without requiring the patient to spend the night in the hospital. Arthroscopic knee surgery is one example. The point is to save money.

Death Spiral: An economics term describing what happens when a health insurance plan becomes hopelessly entrapped in the economic burden of covering an unusually sick patient population. Such a plan is said to be in a death spiral, unable to keep pace with the abnormally high costs of late-stage illness. See **Adverse Selection**.

Defensive Medicine: The massive number of unneces-

sary tests and treatments ordered up by doctors who fear
that if anything goes wrong, they will be accused of doing
less than they should have done and will be sued for malpractice. Medical schools offer courses in malpractice
avoidance, which encourage defensive medicine.

Diagnosis: A judgment by a physician as to the specific nature of a patient's condition.

Diagnosis Related Groups (DRGs): A price-control system devised by Congress that classified all inpatient hospital services rendered under Medicare according to the
patient's main diagnosis and certain other factors. Each
DRG is assigned a fee. Hospitals that take care of the patient for less than the DRG make a profit on the case;
otherwise, they take a loss.

Diagnostic Imaging: Tests, including X-rays, MRIs, and
catheterizations, that provide pictures of a patient's internal organs or physical processes to expand the doctor's
understanding of the person's condition.

Discharge Planning: What hospitals do to prepare for
your departure. Generally, the idea is to get you out
sooner and save money by planning ahead. If a patient
recovering from surgery lives alone, for example, the
hospital may need to order an ambulance to take him
home. If not, the hospital does not want to incur the cost
of an ambulance or an extra day in the hospital just because someone forgot to tell the family to come get him.
Discharge planners also discuss outside rehabilitation facilities with patients, help chronically ill patients to arrange for home health aides or visiting nurses, and
generally try to get the patients out of the hospital before
the treatment moves from the profit to the loss column.

Discount Off Charges: A physician paid in fee-for-service
fashion agrees to give a regular discount, usually 20 percent, to a managed-care plan.

Disenroll: Quit. A Clinton term for an individual's decision to withdraw from an undesirable health plan and join another one.

Downcoding: And you thought all doctors were greedy. Under this accounting procedure, a doctor underplays the value of a medical service, describing it on insurance forms as a simpler procedure than it was, by selecting numerical codes that will yield a lower level of reimbursement. This practice is used mostly by doctors who would not benefit directly from a higher reimbursement, such as group practice physicians or doctors working in managed-care systems. Some say they are saving time on the paperwork by choosing a code that they know is within the range of acceptable services, rather than trying to figure out a more expensive way to report the treatment. Others say they are trying to avoid being accused of inflating the cost of medical care. See **Upcoding**.

Drive-Through Clinics: Doc-in-the-box medicine, from California, of course. Drive up to the service window and roll up your sleeve to get a vaccination or a flu shot. Other simple services provided with similar dispatch. Which means that people seek treatment they might otherwise find too inconvenient and thus stay healthier, while the clinics can save money by delivering services in a more efficient fashion.

ECU (External Care Unit): Hospital slang, black humor for a hopeless case. As in, "Nothing more we can do. Send him to **ECU**."

Employee Tax Cap: The notion of limiting the tax-free status of the health benefits that workers are given by their employers. If a national law is passed mandating universal coverage and a standard benefits package, proponents of managed competition believe that the value of any additional benefits offered by employers should be taxed as personal income.

Employer Mandate: A law requiring employers to pay for health coverage for their workers. Generally, such coverage is also meant to cover the worker's dependents.

Encounter: An actual meeting between a patient and a doctor at which medical service is given. Health plans measure their cost-effectiveness, in part, by limiting the average number and length of encounters. Top HMOs aim to keep those meetings to twelve minutes or less.

Enhancements: Bonuses paid under a performance-based compensation plan for physicians in a managed-care plan, intended to cut costs by curbing treatment. Doctors who follow strict guidelines for treating their patients, such as when to do an angioplasty or order an MRI, can earn a 10 percent bonus or more at the end of the year.

Enrollment: Membership in a health plan.

Enterprise Liability: A system of malpractice litigation favored by the Clinton White House, under which plaintiffs would sue the health-care plan, rather than simply suing the physician accused of malpractice. Proponents maintain that such a system would force physicians to police one another more closely once they were liable for one another's performance and would therefore promote quality. But opponents call it the American Bar Association Full Employment Act. They argue that it would encourage a new storm of litigation under the Deep Pockets principle of law: the bigger and richer the target, the more eagerly personal injury lawyers will pursue it. The Clinton plan requires experimentation with enterprise liability under rules to be devised by the new National Health Board.

Equity: Fairness. As such, it is in the eye of the beholder. Eliminating tax breaks for the generous health coverage enjoyed by corporate employees is one interpretation. Guaranteeing that the poorest American gets precisely the same medical services as the richest one is another.

Exclusions: In insurance, anything the insurer declines to cover. Just as home insurance can exclude earthquake damage, health insurance can exclude skydiving injuries, certain expensive diseases, or other causes for seeking medical care.

Exclusive Providers Organization: An arrangement under which people are allowed to use only a certain group of doctors or hospitals picked by their health plan or their employer.

Experience Rating: The common insurance practice of setting premiums based on the established cost of caring for the insured group in question. Under experience rating, small groups can suffer catastrophic premium increases when one person becomes seriously ill, since one person's high costs can significantly expand the group's total bill.

Family Physician: A doctor who has passed the boards of the American Academy of Family Physicians and has demonstrated proficiency in the full range of general medical skills, from delivering babies to caring for the elderly.

Fee-for-Service: A long-standing practice under which a doctor is paid separate fees for the various medical services provided, from examining a patient or administering a simple test to visiting a patient in the hospital or performing surgery. Critics claim that this practice has encouraged doctors to practice wasteful medicine in order to earn higher reimbursement. Managed care is gradually curbing it.

Fee Schedule: Price controls. A negotiated series of prices for various services that a doctor provides. Government insurance programs impose fee schedules. The Clinton plan would give alliances the power to impose them. See **Resource-Based Relative Value Scale**.

Flexible Benefit Plans: A cost-control measure pioneered by corporations in response to employee demand for new kinds of benefits. Under this type of plan, employees choose from a menu of possible benefits, trading off some guarantees to make room for others.

Flexible Spending Account: Pork-barrel tax reform, circa 1986. Each year, employees can set up these personal accounts, which are funded by payroll deductions. The worker then draws upon the account, using pretax income to pay his or her share of the costs of health services, including deductibles, copayments, and the cost of items like prescription eyeglasses or dental care that may not be covered under the company benefit plan. But allowable items also include many things that can hardly be described as medically necessary, from wigs purchased for purely cosmetic purposes to the costs of some personal litigation. The more a worker spends, the less taxable income is reported. Thus all taxpayers subsidize this open-ended personal spending, which amounts to about $30 billion per year. Congress is expected to eliminate this benefit soon to recapture those 30 billion tax dollars.

Formularies: A list of acceptable prescription drugs approved for use in a health plan and dispensed in its pharmacies. Often, cost-conscious hospitals and health plans exclude very expensive drugs from their formularies. When two moderately priced drugs are roughly equivalent in effectiveness, even if the more costly one works better, the institution may include only the cheaper one on its list. Pharmaceutical manufacturers are spooked by talk of national or regional formularies, which could knock many drugs right off the market.

For-Profit Hospitals, Insurance Companies, Health Plans: This rather awkward phrasing is used to describe investor-owned health entities that attempt to make profits for their shareholders, whether or not they succeed.

Futile Care: Medical care which can do little or nothing to extend life or improve the quality of life. Largely a matter of judgment as to when it begins, futile care is what doctors and hospitals provide when, no matter what they do, the patient will die soon.

Gate Keeper: An employee of a health plan or insurance company, usually a doctor or a nurse, whose job is to make sure that the plan does not spend too much money taking care of patients. Typically, gate keepers discourage referral of patients to expensive specialists. In other cases, they work the phones, asking private physicians why they gave that test, why they want to hospitalize that patient, why they think that patient needs to see a specialist, before approving payment. See **Bean Counter**.

General Practitioner: Anyone who has graduated from medical school and describes his or her practice as general. A GP has not necessarily completed a residency and does not necessarily have the full range of skills that, for example, a family physician is certified to have. Many GPs, though, are part-time specialists who prefer family practice.

Generics: Once a patent expires for a brand-name drug, other companies can market generic versions. Generics are often cheaper. They usually work about as well as the branded equivalent. The generic industry has boomed as insurers have pressed doctors and pharmacists to substitute them for the higher-priced brands and as patients have gained confidence in these lesser-known brand names. Many health plans require generics when available. Nearly half of all prescription drugs sold in the United States are generics.

Global Budget: An overblown term for a national health plan budget that would absolutely limit total medical spending. Borrowed from Canada, embraced by the Clinton White House. The Clinton plan requires states and alliances to control spending by setting per capita insurance premiums, which is a way of setting a health budget and dividing it by the number of people it covers to figure out what they should pay for insurance. The plan also gives alliances the power to reduce physician and health plan fees if it looks as if the annual budget will be exceeded.

Gomer: California hospital slang. As in "He's a **Gomer**." Stands for: Get Out of My Emergency Room. An inside term used among hospital emergency room personnel to identify people they do not want around, such as elderly people asking for help with chronic problems. **Gomers**, they feel, are not their department.

Group Coverage: Any insurance policy that covers a large number of people. Corporations offer group coverage, for example. Generally, these policies are available at better prices because the costs of providing health services are spread over a larger number of people, many of whom are very healthy.

Group Practice: An organization of doctors who jointly offer their services, often in the form of a corporation, typically in or near a particular hospital. Kaiser Permanente is the oldest and largest group practice, employing about ten thousand doctors.

Health Alliances: A basic building block of President Clinton's health-reform proposal, these are large purchasers of health services that represent virtually everyone in a given state or region. Very large companies may be permitted not to join.

Health Card: President Clinton's idea for a medical identification card for every American that would ease access to health services.

Health Care: A broad reference to all of the medical and other health services a person might want or need to maintain good health. As distinguished from medical care, health care may include hygienic, nutritional, therapeutic, or other matters that do not involve medical professionals.

Health Insurance Purchasing Cooperative (HIPC, pronounced *hippick*): Another term for a health alliance, HIPCs are an element of the managed-competition model. These entities would buy health services for large groups of people in a given region by making contracts with health-care plans.

Health Maintenance Organization (HMO): This type of health-care plan covers all needed medical services for a prepaid, usually monthly, fee and minimizes copayments. The idea is to make it cheaper to stay healthy. But some HMOs are still a lot better at holding down costs than they are at providing quality care.

Health Provider Shortage Area: White House term for an area that has too few doctors and nurses and is targeted for assistance.

Health Security: You can get medical help when you need it, and you will have adequate coverage for the costs.

Heels on Wheels: A law enforcement term for con artists who operate portable clinics to perpetrate large-scale Medicaid fraud.

High-Risk Pools: An insurance term that describes a group of insured people who are likelier than the average person to need costly medical help. Elderly, chronically ill, and disabled people are typical of high-risk pools, as are the inner-city poor, who are more vulnerable to health problems related to poor nutrition, high blood pressure, drug abuse, and violent crime.

Holistic Care: A nontraditional approach to treatment, usually employing a lot of methods that are not sanctioned by the American Medical Association or based in accepted scientific fact. See **Alternative Medicine.**

Home Care: Medical or custodial services provided in the patient's home.

Home Health Aide: A person who helps an ailing person at home, whether in bathing, dressing, cooking, or cleaning. Generally this service is used by people recovering from surgery, people with chronic illness, or disabled or elderly people who would otherwise be forced to move into a custodial or nursing facility because they cannot handle all of their basic needs without assistance. Not to be confused with skilled nursing care. See **Visiting Nurse**.

Hospice: A facility that cares for the terminally ill.

Hospital Affiliation: An agreement under which a hospital contracts to provide inpatient services to members of a health plan.

Hospital Privileges: Arrangements under which doctors are allowed to treat their patients in a particular hospital. An obstetrician, for example, delivers babies in a hospital where he has privileges. Many family physicians complain that the only reason they cannot perform certain services for their patients is that the hospitals reserve those privileges for specialists. They argue that this deprives them of income and costs their patients more, since they must consult other doctors to gain access to tests and procedures.

Imaging: Any number of noninvasive diagnostic procedures, from X-rays to MRIs, that yield pictures of a patient's internal organs and functions so that doctors can better understand their condition.

Inappropriate Care: Medical treatment that may not be necessary and for which the medical risk exceeds the likely medical benefit to the patient. Unnecessary surgery, for example.

Indemnity: A form of insurance that reimburses patients

for all services covered under the policy. Because patients with indemnity coverage have more latitude in their choice of medical services than do patients in closely managed health plans like HMOs, indemnity coverage is usually more expensive.

Individual Practice Association (IPA): A medical middleman. An IPA agrees to provide medical services to patients for a negotiated fee. The IPA then contracts with individual physicians, who continue in their private practice or separate group practices but treat the IPA clients on a fee-for-service, price-controlled, or per capita basis.

Inpatient Care: Medical treatment given to hospitalized patients. The trick is to make it outpatient care, to try to avoid the greater expense of treating them in hospitals.

Insurer: Can be almost anyone these days. Insurance companies used to be financial entities that managed risk for large numbers of people. These days, lots of new faces are insurers, including employers, doctors, IPOs, hospitals, managed-care companies, and other organizations. Even as this evolution has occurred, many insurance companies have been reaching beyond risk management to manage health plans and then to offer their own health plans, HMOs, and other medical services.

Integrated Health Network: They're springing up everywhere. Johns Hopkins in Baltimore, the New York Hospital, Intermountain Health Care in Salt Lake City, the Mayo Clinic, and Northwestern Medical in Chicago to name a few. A local health services conglomerate, usually built around a major hospital that offers cradle-to-grave medical care. Typically, these networks link hospitals, outpatient clinics, community medical centers, health maintenance organizations, and other services with a large pool of physicians. In some cases, the network also offers its own insurance plan and has informal relationships with physicians' groups in outlying areas. If Congress enacts a health-reform law based on the managed-competition model, these vertically integrated networks will be ready to compete and may be large enough to service state health alliances. But even without federal reform, these networks are very competitive, generally of very high quality, and are proliferating. See **Managed Competition**.

Intermediate-Care Facility: Less than a hospital, more than room and board. Includes some nursing homes and rehabilitation facilities.

Jackson Hole Group: The inventors of managed competition. A private think tank dominated by insurance companies, hospital groups, and large corporations that meets periodically at the home of Dr. Paul Ellwood, its founder, in Jackson Hole, Wyoming, to discuss ways of improving health services. Participants include Blue Cross/Blue Shield, Aetna, Cigna, the Prudential, Metropolitan Life, General Motors, General Electric, the American Medical Association, U.S. Healthcare, PacifiCare, Columbia / HCA Healthcare, the Sisters of Providence Hospital System, Glaxo, Pfizer, and the Mayo Clinic.

Job Lock: What happens when an individual is afraid to change jobs for fear of losing health insurance.

Long-Term Care: Extended assistance for chronically ill, mentally ill, and disabled people, which in its best form seeks to make them as independent as possible. Often focused primarily on assistance with carrying out basic daily needs. This term also describes what nursing homes provide. The long-term-care industry is growing rapidly as the American population ages. Already, one in four Americans either suffers from chronic illness or is responsible for taking care of a family member who does.

Long-Term-Care Coverage: Insurance designed to meet the needs of the disabled, mentally ill, and chronically ill so that they do not have to depend upon friends and relatives for help or on Medicaid.

Magnetic Resonance Imager (MRI): A sophisticated diagnostic-imaging machine that produces clear pictures of the patient's internal organs. MRI is also a reference to the test conducted using such a machine.

Malpractice: A judgment that a doctor or other health provider has caused a patient injury because of sloppy, botched, or inadequate treatment.

Malpractice Reform: Calls for changes in the legal system that would reduce the number of dubious lawsuits against doctors, as well as the costs of the litigation. Tort reform is a necessary part of any scheme to control overall health costs, since fear of malpractice leads to defensive medicine, and the skyrocketing premiums for malpractice insurance are forcing doctors to stop practicing in critical specialties such as obstetrics. The Clinton plan offers doctors very little help here and defines a consumer's right to sue not only a physician but an alliance, a state alliance authority, and even the Secretary of Health and Human Services in some cases. See **Enterprise Liability**.

Managed Care: Any health delivery system in which someone in charge of paying the bills can second-guess decisions made by doctors or patients on the kinds of medical services provided. Managed-care organizations, such as HMOs, group practices, and insurance-managed health plans, seek to control costs by curbing excessive use of tests, hospitalization, visits to specialists, and other services.

Managed Competition: The number one oxymoron of health-care policy. A health-care system that attempts to give consumers better service by consolidating their buying power and promoting competition among providers such as doctors, hospitals, and HMOs. Under this model, the government sets certain basic standards — such as universal coverage, portable benefits, and quality standards — that all health-care plans must meet. Purchasing cooperatives, also called alliances, buy health services for those who live in a given area by negotiating contracts with providers. (Very large companies might be allowed to arrange their own separate health services.) The cooperatives wield considerable market power, since they represent so many people. Doctors and hospitals would probably form organized groups (health-care plans) to compete for the business. See **Integrated Health Network**.

Managed Cooperation: An apt term that President Clinton adopted for his proposal after some economists complained that his approach to health-care reform was not really a managed-competition plan. The Clinton plan closely regulates competition, requiring plenty of cooperation with government officials.

Managed Regulation: How doctors describe the Clinton plan.

Mandated Benefits: The package of benefits that everyone is guaranteed. See **Employer Mandate**.

Mandated Providers: The types of skilled medical professionals — possibly including specialists and psychiatrists — whose services must be included under the requirements of a given plan.

Marketing Restrictions: The Clinton term for the plan's new rules tightly regulating the advertising and marketing of health services.

Medicaid: A federal-state insurance program that attempts to cover the poor and the impoverished elderly.

Medicaid Mills: Fly-by-night storefront operations that purport to treat Medicaid patients but usually specialize in narcotics trading and Medicaid fraud.

Medical Care: Not the same as health care, this term describes medical services given to a patient by a doctor, nurse, or hospital. Generally, it describes medical help when a patient is ill or has been injured, as well as diagnostic supervision and treatment of chronic conditions. See **Health Care.**

Medicare: A federal program that finances medical care for the elderly and some disabled Americans.

Medigap Insurance: A stop-gap policy that covers payment of a Medicare beneficiary's share of medical costs, as well as certain medical services, such as prescription drugs, that are not yet covered under Medicare.

Menu: Sometimes used to describe information about the health plans among which consumers would choose under a managed-competition system. In the Cooper plan, the menu, provided by the alliance, spells out the health plans available, the prices that consumers would pay to use them, and information about the quality of the plans and summaries of consumer satisfaction surveys conducted among people who use each plan. See similar term, **Report Card.**

National Council on Graduate Medical Education: A new regulatory office proposed by the Clinton plan. Created within the Health and Human Services agency and run by the HHS secretary, the council would dictate the number and types of openings in graduate medical schools. In addition to deciding how many students could specialize, say, in gastroenterology versus cardiology, the council would allocate openings in these schools based on targets for regulating the number of doctors in particular specialties who are members of racial and ethnic minorities.

National Health Board: A powerful new federal agency, proposed by the Clinton White House, that would regulate the practice of medicine and the provision of health benefits by the states and would have broad legal authority in the resolution of claims by health consumers. Among other things, the board will devise the national health budget, decide what constitutes medical necessity, define the benefits guaranteed to all Americans, decide whether to add new required benefits, and in numerous other ways regulate health care in the United States. Using data on the results of operations and other procedures, for example, the board could make rules about when an operation should be done or when certain tests would be permitted. The board will also try to make sure that, according to rules it devises, no state spends too much or too little providing health-care services.

Negligence: The doctor's nightmare. In medicine, a legal term describing a judgment that a physician or other provider has hurt a patient by failing to provide complete, competent, and watchful care.

Network: Any group of doctors and/or hospitals that jointly provide care to a given group of patients covered by a health-care plan. Typically, these networks offer discounts to win the business. Their advantage is convenience — the network offers a broad range of health services.

No-Fault System: A concept borrowed from other areas of litigation, from no-fault auto insurance to no-fault divorces, no-fault malpractice has never really caught on. Enterprise liability, the strangely named White House concept, embodies the spirit of no-fault. See **Enterprise Liability**.

Noneconomic Losses: In malpractice, the portion of the legal judgment that is awarded to compensate for losses that cannot directly be measured in dollars, such as pain and suffering.

Nonoverlapping Networks: In some markets, the same doctors work for competing health plans. But in nonoverlapping networks, a doctor who serves patients in one plan is not allowed to serve patients in another, whether he is a salaried employee of a plan or a private practitioner. Private practitioners often are forced to surrender their independence in order to gain access to enough patients. See **Closed Panel**.

Nonphysician Practitioners: Surprise. They're not doctors. This clunky term refers to nurses and others who provide treatment. They know less, and they cost less.

Not-for-Profit Hospitals, Clinics, HMOs, etc.: Healthcare institutions that spend whatever profits they may make on providing the services they offer, rather than paying them to shareholders, as investor-owned institutions do. As such, not-for-profits typically call their profits "excess revenues."

Nurse: A licensed medical professional who has completed a recognized course of nursing training. Generally speaking, nurses cannot prescribe medicine or perform surgery and usually follow a plan of treatment laid out by a physician. Providing services ranging from simple compassionate care to sophisticated monitoring of critical illness, nurses are the hospital patient's main link to medical help and often save lives as a result.

Nurse Practitioner: A nurse with advanced training who typically can prescribe some medications and counsel patients on a course of treatment without consulting a physician.

Open Access: An insurance term describing the right of a patient to decide to see a specialist without seeking anyone's approval, though that specialist must usually be a designated member of the health plan's provider list.

Open Enrollment: A requirement that anyone can apply for coverage by a particular health plan. Under a managed-competition plan, people would have the opportunity to change health plans during an open enrollment period once a year.

Outcomes Analysis: Quality research in medicine that seeks to learn how patients fare after treatment, as a way of improving medical practice. The relatively new field of outcomes research is slowly building a knowledge base about what really works in medicine by monitoring millions of patient cases and analyzing the long-term results of their treatment.

Outcomes Management: What doctors and health officials can do once they have better data on the results of medical treatment and therefore on what works best. They will be able to manage the outcomes themselves by pursuing the best course of treatment in the first place. Outcomes management is an organized system of improving quality in medical care.

Out-of-Pocket Costs: The share of medical costs the patient must pay.

Outpatient Treatment: Medical care that does not require a night's stay in the hospital. Hospitals provide such care in outpatient clinics, some of which are located on hospital grounds.

Overlapping Networks: Medical markets where doctors are free to join a number of health plans, some of which compete with one another. Under such a system, a particular physician may care for patients in more than one plan and be paid at different rates. See **Nonoverlapping Networks**.

Package Pricing: A method of compensating hospitals under which a standard package rate is charged for all treatment associated with a given procedure, such as a heart transplant or bypass. The idea is to pressure the doctors and hospital administrators to reconsider tests, extra days in the hospital, and other costly elements associated with the procedure, since they will lose money if they provide too much treatment under the controlled price.

Parity: What the other guy is getting. Often used by mental health providers to demand coverage of the full range of services they offer, from talk therapy to psychiatric hospitalization, in parity with comprehensive medical benefits that range from preventive care to hospitalization. This term is also used by AARP to argue that any benefit in President Clinton's proposed universal coverage package must be included under the Medicare plan even if the Medicare plan offers other benefits that are not included in the package everyone else is getting.

Part-Timer: The Clinton plan defines this as someone who works between 40 and 120 hours per month for a firm. Part-timers will be eligible to receive full health benefits. The employer and the taxpayers will divide the cost, depending on how many hours the person works.

Pay or Play: As a presidential candidate, Bill Clinton endorsed this plan before he discovered managed competition. A national health system under which all employers would be required either to "play" (i.e., provide health insurance for their workers), or else "pay" the government a set fee to do so.

Peer Review: The system by which medical professionals review the work of their colleagues, probing for flaws, as an adjunct to cutting hospital costs.

Peer Review Organizations (PROs): Entities responsible for evaluating the quality of treatment offered by physicians. PROs also consider, before or after the fact, whether decisions to hospitalize patients are warranted. These organizations are responsible for lowering hospital admission rates where possible as a cost-control measure, while guarding against shoddy care.

Per Capita Target: Under the Clinton plan, projected health budgets for states or regional alliances would be expressed in terms of targeted spending per capita.

Personal Physician: An archaic term denoting an era in which most people had family doctors and actually knew them. These days, a personal physician can be anyone from a general practitioner to a urologist or cardiologist or a neurosurgeon, if that is the doctor the patient knows and trusts.

Phantom Visits: One way that some doctors abuse the insurance honor system. They bill insurance companies for visiting their patients in the hospital, when they actually did not. Hard to monitor, since people in the hospital are usually too sick to be certain who came by.

Physical Therapy (PT): Special exercise to make sick people stronger, covered on a limited outpatient basis in the president's plan. PT can range from mouth exercises to help stroke victims regain the ability to enunciate to massage and supervised stretching exercises for people recovering from major surgery to assistance in relearning how to perform the most rudimentary physical actions after a serious injury.

Physician Groups: Any organization of physicians for the purpose of serving patients. See **Group Practice**.

Physician-Hospital Organization (PHO): A health plan under which patients get all of their medical treatment from the doctors and hospitals in the group. The PHO provides the insurance, too, eliminating insurance companies and HMOs as middlemen.

Playing the Doctor: What thieves do when they operate Medicaid mills, pretending to provide medical services as a front for drug-dealing and Medicaid fraud. See **Medicaid Mills**.

Playing Robin Hood: A commonly used term for what hospitals do when they charge the well insured higher prices in order to obtain funds for training, treatment of the uninsured poor, and other services. They rob the rich. That's one reason why a Bufferin tablet can cost $5 in a hospital. See **Cross-Subsidizing**.

Point of Enrollment (POE) Plan: A health-care plan that

offers a choice when people enroll: either they can sign up for the lower-cost, tightly managed part of the plan, usually an HMO, or they can pay more to retain the option of using doctors and hospitals that are not included in the HMO.

Point of Service (POS) Plan: More flexible than point of enrollment plans. In this model, people decide whenever they need medical help (at the point of service) whether to see the providers authorized by the closely managed part of the plan — usually an HMO — or to pay more to choose another doctor or hospital. They can change their minds from month to month, from illness to illness. By leaving the door open on future decisions, this model encourages people to use the lower-cost, managed-care part of the plan. If they develop a serious illness, they have the option of seeing the doctors they choose. Included in the Clinton plan, except if a state or alliance decides to be a single-payer system.

Practice Standards: To improve the quality of medical care, researchers seek to learn enough about what works best to devise some general guidelines for doctors on how to treat each kind of condition. These guidelines are called practice standards.

Preadmission Certification: Patients (or their doctors) must check with the bean counters at the insurance company before the patient is admitted to the hospital. Regardless of medical need, some insurance plans will not pay the bills if this procedure is not followed.

Preexisting Conditions: Health conditions the person had before the insurance coverage took effect, whether or not they knew it, and which the insurer therefore declines responsibility for covering. Examples can range from a woman who becomes pregnant before obtaining insurance to a person with AIDS or cancer who does not reveal that information to the insurer when obtaining coverage. In recent years, the term has taken on sinister overtones as insurance companies have applied it in abusive and, often, intrusive ways to justify dropping coverage for individuals or whole companies. Some insurers, for example, covertly tested new applicants' blood samples for HIV and other signs of trouble. Others increased the qualifiers in policies, refusing to cover a wide variety of conditions that were vaguely linked to prior health habits or problems and that might lead to costly medical treatment. See **Exclusions**.

Preferred Provider Organization (PPO): Something like an HMO, this is a group of doctors, sometimes also hospitals, which offers a form of prepaid coverage. Usually the group has offered a discount to a company to lock in the business of treating its employees.

Preferred Providers: Are they better than ordinary providers? No. They are the doctors or hospitals that your employer or health plan has chosen to treat you.

Pregnancy-Related Services: Birth control or medical services provided to women who are pregnant. Some people use this term as a euphemism for abortion, especially when explaining that the services are covered in the president's plan.

Premiums: Traditionally, the fee paid for health coverage, usually to insurance companies. More recently, in an attempt to avoid the T-word, the Clinton administration has adopted this term to describe new kinds of payroll taxes that would finance health coverage.

Prepaid Health Plan: A health system under which all necessary medical services are provided for a pre-set fee. Health maintenance organizations are typical prepaid plans.

Preventive Care: A vague term for medical care that aims to avoid serious illness by enabling doctors to spot trouble early during checkups. Essentially, services like well-baby exams, physicals, and mammograms that monitor basic health status.

Primary Care: This term, a favorite of managed-care companies, has no medical definition. Sometimes it is little more than a euphemism for basic care with limited access to specialists. It does not necessarily mean treatment by physicians or even nurses.

Primary Care Doctor: Everybody wants to be one, because under managed care, which limits access to secondary treatment by specialists, the primary care doctor always gets paid. The patients are the commodity. Specialists call themselves primary care doctors in order to build regular relationships with patients and ensure themselves a reliable stream of revenue.

Primary Health Care: As defined in the Clinton legislation, primary health care includes family medicine, general internal medicine, pediatrics, obstetrics, and gynecology. Under the Clinton plan, the federal government would require that at least 55 percent of all medical school graduates are trained primary care physicians. In 1993, about 45 percent of practicing physicians fit that definition, but far fewer medical students intended to enter those fields.

Private Pay: You pay.

Private Practice: This term refers to physicians who are basically small business owners who take care of a certain group of regular patients. They may be family doctors or specialists. Other physicians, such as the members of group practices or the salaried employees of health maintenance organizations, agree to help cover a larger population of people and often do not know their patients.

Prospective Budget: The maximum that the government or alliance plans to spend on health care in the coming year.

Prospective Payment: A form of price controls, this is what the government is willing to pay for a medical service.

Provider: A hospital, health maintenance organization, doctor, or anyone else who offers medical services. Usually this term is limited to those who must be licensed by the states.

Provider Cartels: Think OPEC. Situations where doctors and hospitals, working together, lock up enough of the local market so that they are able to charge exorbitantly high rates for lack of competition.

Purchasing Cooperatives: An element of the managed-competition model for health systems, these are farmers markets of medicine that buy health services for a large group of individuals by negotiating contracts with health plans. As transformed in the president's plan, the co-ops are far larger and more powerful; he calls them **Alliances**, which see.

Qualifying Employee: A Clinton plan term for an employee who works at least forty hours per month for a company and is therefore eligible to be covered as an employee of that firm. See **Part-Timer**.

Quality: In medicine, quality is the right diagnosis and treatment delivered promptly and competently. Since costs go down as medical quality improves, quality is also measured by efficiency.

Quality Health Care: Means different things to different people. In medicine, it generally means the best and most effective care that doctors know how to provide. But in political parlance, budget constraints and political judgments about fairness change the meaning of the term. Quality then usually means that no one gets more than anyone else and that the care is the best that the system can afford to provide. In a tightly budgeted health-care system, such as the one envisioned by President Clinton, it is not at all clear that the best care available would be the best that medicine knows how to provide.

Quality Waste: This economics term, used by hospital

managers and researchers, describes the amount of waste in medical systems that is caused by sloppy procedures or bad planning and which is reduced when overall quality improves. If a doctor does a poor job in surgery, for example, the patient may have to spend more time recovering in the hospital (wasting unnecessary days of expensive care), or may even need another operation. If a patient is given a diagnostic test that was not called for, the test is quality waste. Quality waste includes incorrect diagnoses and unnecessary medications, as well as such mundane items as excessive use of disposable hospital supplies or inefficient discharge planning that causes patients to spend unnecessary additional days in the hospital when they could have gone home earlier.

Rationing: When medical resources are not adequate to meet demand, providers ration care, deciding who gets what. In its milder forms, this is a way of saving money by eliminating things that people can do without. But judgments about what is really needed become more difficult to make when financial pressures become severe. Rationing then can mean that older people are not given lifesaving operations or that other patients cannot receive services that doctors believe they need. If American health costs rise to untenable levels, rationing is certain to grow more intensive.

Redundant Care: Unnecessary medical treatment or tests that merely duplicate other findings, contributing nothing of significance.

Referral Loop: The process by which a family doctor refers patients to specialists for certain problems, then expects the specialists to refer the patient back to the family doctor for general care.

Rehabilitation: The branch of medicine that specializes in restoring injured or crippled patients to the fullest possible health and strength, largely through physical therapy.

Report Card: A managed competition idea included in the president's proposal. Health plans would be given report cards that would measure how well they served their patients. Consumers choosing a plan offered by their purchasing alliance would be able to judge the providers not only on price but also on quality and patient satisfaction. Provider report cards would measure performance in such areas as their immunization rate, the percentage of pregnant women who received certain kinds of prenatal treatment, the survival rate for heart bypass surgery, or even whether dissatisfied patients quit the plan. See **Accountability**.

Resource-Based Relative Value Scale (RBRVS): A price-regulating formula devised by Medicare under which doctors and other providers are reimbursed according to their training and skill, while also taking into account their overhead costs and the amount of service they give. The goal is to pay family doctors more, since they spend more time with patients and play a critical role in preventing serious illness, and to pay surgeons and specialists less. One hospital chairman jokes that for his prestigious institution, where most of the physicians are specialists, RBRVS means "Real Bad Revenue Very Soon."

Risk: The formula under which insurance companies balance the anticipated expense of covering medical treatment for their beneficiaries against their ability to recover those costs through premiums and investments.

Risk Avoidance: The efforts by insurers to minimize their financial obligations to beneficiaries by avoiding generous benefits, costly treatment, and sicker people. See **Preexisting Conditions**.

Risk-Bonus Arrangements: In about one-third of all HMOs, the specialists share the financial risk of patient coverage, and their bonus is tied to budget targets. This means that if they spend more treating their patients, they may earn markedly less. Some plans hold back 20 percent of a doctor's annual pay unless he comes in on budget.

Rural Problem: A phrase used to describe a natural limitation of the managed-competition model, which probably would not work well in sparsely populated areas with few doctors and, therefore, little potential for price competition among health plans.

Secondary Care: Treatment by specialists, usually upon referral by the patient's family physician, who is described as providing primary care.

Self-Referral: An unethical practice under which doctors order services for their patients from laboratories or other medical facilities in which they have a direct financial interest, usually without disclosing this conflict of interest to the patient. The facility may be a diagnostic imaging center, a blood lab, a hospital, a group practice, or a joint venture of some kind. Although forms of this practice have been outlawed in some states and discouraged by numerous medical societies, it is still common.

Sentinel Effect: The tendency by some physicians to order fewer tests and procedures than might be wise, because they anticipate criticism from their gate keepers or other financial minders. Generally seen in HMOs and group practices that closely monitor each doctor's treatment costs.

Shadow Pricing: A way for a discount supplier to maximize profits while protecting a price advantage. Retailers do it, and so do HMOs and profit-making hospitals. While they raise their prices at the same rate as their competitors do, charging essentially what the market will bear, they are careful to stay just behind the high-priced health plan or in its shadow. Thus they seem to be operating more efficiently because their prices are always a little lower.

Sicker and Quicker: Medical slang for the all-too-common hospital practice of releasing patients too soon, sometimes before they are stable, in order to save money.

Single-Form System: Hillary Rodham Clinton's term for a system in which all providers would use the same insurance form. See **Single-Payer System.**

Single-Payer State, Alliance: Under the Clinton plan, an alliance could operate as a single-payer system and limit consumer health choices while closely regulating health services. A state could declare itself to be a single-payer system and impose a single, state-run health plan. See **Single-Payer System.**

Single-Payer System: A centrally controlled health system in which all payments for medical care are issued from a single source, the government. The government gets the money by raising taxes. Canada has such a system. While people in Canada can choose their own doctors, the government regulates all aspects of health care, controls spending, levies high taxes to finance it, pays the bills, and cuts benefits when money is tight. Many members of the Clinton administration health staff said they thought the United States should set up a national single-payer system. The Clinton plan shares many features with such an economic structure, including complex price controls, extensive new federal and local regulation of medicine, and an option for states to become single-payer systems.

Sin Taxes: Special taxes levied on products such as cigarettes and alcoholic beverages to support social programs. Generally, the assumption is that people who indulge in certain habits have an obligation to pay more for health or other programs. The Clinton plan relies on a sin tax of 75 cents per pack on cigarettes. The administration strongly considered additional sin taxes on alcoholic beverages and guns and ammunition.

Skilled Nursing Facility: Certified by Medicare, these institutions must provide such designated services as twenty-four-hour nursing and physical, occupational, and speech therapy.

Small Group Reform: The idea of changing the way insurance companies set premiums for individuals and small groups, charging them much higher prices than large groups must pay. All of the leading proposals for national health reform include this idea.

Specialist: The typical American doctor, this is a physician who has pursued advanced training in a particular area of medicine, such as ophthalmology or urology, and usually limits his or her practice to that area. Even a family physician is a specialist, since the necessary range of skills to adequately practice family medicine have been defined and must be certified by the American Academy of Family Physicians.

Specialty Capitation: A group of specialists serving an HMO or other managed health plan agrees to accept a per capita fee (annual budget) for treating a group of patients, regardless of how much care the patients actually need. This is a direct financial incentive to withhold treatment.

Spend Down: Impoverish oneself in order to qualify for Medicaid coverage. In order to get help with their nursing-home costs, for example, many Medicare patients must spend down to poverty levels before they are entitled to Medicaid coverage.

Step Care: What you need, as you need it. Generally, this describes residential complexes in which elderly or chronically ill people can live in private homes or apartments as long as they are able and can then move into another part of the complex for skilled nursing assistance when they progress to a point where they need those kinds of services. Preferred by many elderly people because it gives them the opportunity to preserve their independence as long as possible in something resembling a community setting, while secure in the knowledge that medical help and home health services are available when necessary.

Step-Down Unit: A special hospital ward for patients who are well enough to leave intensive care but still in need of closer supervision than they would get in a regular hospital room.

Supplementary Coverage: Any insurance that bridges a gap between major coverage and medical need. Often refers to the special policies that AARP sells to the elderly to fill gaps in Medicare coverage, such as the costs of medications. AARP is one of the largest sellers of this kind of insurance in the United States.

Taking Assignment: The practice under which doctors agree to accept whatever the insurer will pay, rather than insisting that a patient pay more.

Tax Cap: A limit on the tax deductibility of corporate benefits.

Tertiary Care: Treatment provided by top-level medical professionals with highly specialized skills, including neurosurgeons, thoracic surgeons, and intensive care units. Tertiary care is costly, since these physicians often require a good deal of sophisticated technology and the technicians to run it.

Therapeutic Equivalents: A drug that will work about the same as another drug, as measured by the patient's progress in recovering from illness.

Third-Party Payment: A main reason for explosive U.S. health-care costs, this is the system under which most people expect someone else — an insurer — to pay for their medical care. Third-party systems such as corporate group coverage do enhance access but often tend to encourage unnecessary usage of medical services.

Tort Reform: Reform of the legal system. In medical terms, tort reform is needed to curb the costs of malpractice litigation and defensive medicine.

Triage: A system of prioritizing treatment when a sudden surge of severe medical need overwhelms a hospital or health plan. Doctors triage in wartime. Hospitals triage during natural disasters, treating the most seriously wounded first and leaving the dying and the less-seriously wounded for later. More generally, the state of Oregon has worked out a system of triage for its Medicaid system, deciding which medical conditions will get full coverage and which will not.

Two-Tiered Health-Care System: A system like the one in the United States that does not guarantee that everyone gets precisely the same medical service in exactly the same surroundings. In other words, one where some people can afford to obtain medical services, conveniences, or amenities that others cannot. Blasted as immoral by some, celebrated as emblematic of the American way by others.

Unbundling: Basically, padding the bill. In many cases, doctors and hospitals can earn much higher reimbursement for the services they provide if they "unbundle" the costs, billing separately for each element of the procedure. Some operations, for example, can be described as one procedure (a full hysterectomy), at one price, or several jobs (the removal of the Fallopian tubes, the removal of the ovaries, and so on, plus the routine repair of various things along the way), for a much higher total.

Uncompensated Care: The patient did not pay for it.

Undercompensated Care: The patient or government insurance plan did not pay enough for it, meaning the hospital was paid less than it cost it to provide the medical service. Biggest example: Medicaid.

Undifferentiated Patient: A human being. A person who

has not yet been diagnosed by a doctor and thence classified as a particular medical problem.

Uniformity: A term used often in the health legislation President Clinton submitted to Congress. While the plan purports to give states great latitude in designing health services, it also gives the federal government broad powers to enforce uniformity among health services across the United States.

Universal Access: Not the same as the universal coverage promised under the Clinton plan. Universal access usually means that everybody can find doctors when necessary, though Congressman Jim Cooper uses it to mean that everyone can afford to buy insurance coverage.

Universal Coverage: Everyone is insured.

Unnecessary Care: Medical treatment that will not necessarily help the patient, such as extra tests and procedures with an uncertain benefit. It is not always clear what is necessary and what is not.

Upcoding: Auto repair shops do it, and many doctors do, too. Upcoding is how doctors and hospitals filling out insurance forms pad the bill by exaggerating what they have done. On insurance forms, medical services are assigned numerical codes, and rates of reimbursement are tied to the codes. Pick one code and the insurance company pays a certain amount; but pick the one that describes a more complex service and the insurer pays more. Patients profit, too. Some ordinary doctor visits, such as checkups, are not reimbursed by insurers. But the insurance covers the visit if the doctor exaggerates the condition of the patient. Upcoding is the reason that when you visit your doctor for a mundane problem, you are often horrified by the severity of the terms that describe it on the receipt you are given for your insurance plan. Don't worry. You are not sicker than you thought; your doctor has upcoded you. See, believe it or not, **Downcoding**.

Utilization: The extent to which people use health services.

Utilization Review: A cost-control measure in which a hospital or other supervisory entity formally monitors a physician's practice or a hospital's services to analyze whether patients are getting the right amount of care and whether doctors are overindulging in certain kinds of treatment.

Visiting Nurse: They make house calls! Covered at least in limited fashion under Medicare, Medicaid, and much private insurance, these registered nurses visit the homebound, whether sick or disabled, to provide medical service and monitor their condition.

Voluntary Alliances: The Clinton plan would require every American to join a health alliance. But some states, including Florida and California, already have versions of managed competition in place that permit consumers and small businesses to decide whether they want to join the alliances. Critics say that voluntary alliances will not do enough to spur competition among health plans. Capitol Hill sources say the big insurance companies would never support a national health plan that made the alliances voluntary. Reason: profits would plummet because of **Adverse Selection,** which see.

Voluntary Price Restraints: Some health providers have offered to coordinate voluntary price controls. Clinton officials prefer government price controls. The pharmaceutical industry asked the Clinton Justice Department for permission to coordinate such restraints but was turned down. Doctors have also discussed volunteering such restraints. The Clinton plan includes mechanisms for regulating provider fees as well as drug prices.

Vulnerable Populations: A federal euphemism for poor people. When discussing health reform, it sometimes also means drug addicts and alcoholics.

Well: When used to describe people who had been sick, the word "well" once meant that the patient had recovered from the illness. In the world of managed care, however, "well" is often a euphemism for a budgetary concept. A patient is pronounced "well" when he or she has used up the quota of medical services that the health plan is willing to expend on treatment of the illness.

Wellness: A Yuppie kind of word, like "parenting." We have always had parents, for example, but "parenting" incorporates the notion that there is a better way to be a parent. "Wellness" describes the goal of keeping people well, which is cheaper than treating them when they get sick. Corporations emphasize wellness, as if good health needed a new sales pitch. Embedded in the term is the notion that staying healthy is not a matter of luck or personal choice, that individuals owe the larger group a commitment to the habits that promote good health. Some employers and HMOs offer wellness incentives, giving money or time off to workers who never take sick days or who quit smoking or lose weight or in some other way meet the collective wellness goals.

Which Doctors: Family physicians. As in "which specialist doctor should I send my patient to?" A derisive term used by some medical students, specialists, and medical Pooh-Bahs to describe family doctors, who must rely upon specialists to treat many of their patients' complicated problems.

White Collar Wilding: A term used by prosecutors to describe freewheeling Medicaid fraud committed by well-dressed professionals, usually doctors and lawyers, who have learned how to rip off the system.

Whole Patient: This may sound like a term for someone who has never had an organ removed, but that's not it. The name of a philosophical movement in medicine, this phrase describes a way of thinking about patients in terms of everything that affects their health, with the goal of shaping comprehensive medical services. The philosophy attempts to counter the proclivity of modern medical science to think of patients as specific medical problems, rather than people. Health maintenance organizations were conceived as a way of serving the health needs of the whole patient.

Windfall Profits: In medicine, a judgment that a supplier of health goods or services is making excessive profits. Most frequently applied by critics of insurance companies and drugmakers.

Withhold: The portion of a physician's annual compensation, usually 15 percent or 20 percent, that is held back by the health plan until the end of the year. The doctor earns the "withhold" only if the costs of treating his or her patients — or all patients treated by the group — do not exceed a budget target. Ironically, this term also describes a direct financial incentive to withhold care.

NOTES

Chapter One: Basic Principles

1. "Substance Abuse: The Nation's Number One Health Problem," prepared by the Institute for Health Policy, Brandeis University, for the Robert Wood Johnson Foundation, Princeton, New Jersey, October 1993.
2. Ibid.
3. Ibid.
4. U.S. Department of Transportation, National Highway Traffic Safety Administration.
5. The Children's Aid Society.
6. Ibid.

Chapter Three: Condition: Critical

1. The American Hospital Association.
2. U.S. Health Care Financing Administration.
3. Governor Lawton Chiles, interview, August 1993.
4. U.S. Department of Labor.
5. Employee Benefit Research Institute; U.S. Bureau of the Census, Current Population Survey, March 1993.
6. Robert Blendon, M.D., Harvard School of Public Health.
7. U.S. Department of Health and Human Services.
8. Ibid.
9. James Todd, M.D., executive vice president, American Medical Association, interview, August 1993.
10. U.S. Bureau of the Census.
11. Author interview, September 1993.
12. *Fortune*, June 3, 1991.
13. Commerce Clearing House, Washington, D.C.
14. Author interview, July 1993.
15. American Hospital Association.

16. Lewin/ICF.

17. U.S. Bureau of the Census, Current Population Survey, March 1993.

18. American Medical Association.

19. Kassebaum and Szenas, "Specialty Preferences of Graduating Medical Students: 1992 Update," based on The Association of American Medical Colleges 1992 Graduation Questionnaire, *Journal of the American Medical Association,* September 1, 1993, p. 1070.

20. Data from the 1992 Annual Survey of Graduate Medical Education Programs, American Medical Association, Chicago, Illinois.

21. David A. Kindig, M.D., Ph.D., James M. Cultice, Fitzhugh Mullan, M.D., "The Elusive Generalist Physician: Can We Reach a 50% Goal?" *Journal of the American Medical Association,* September 1, 1993, pp. 1069–73.

22. Ibid., and author interviews, June–September, 1993.

23. General Motors.

24. Milliman & Robertson, health finance consultants.

25. General Motors.

26. Group Health Association of America, December 1993.

27. Group Health Association of America, survey, December 1993.

28. United HealthCare Corporation.

29. National Health Care Anti-Fraud Association.

30. Aetna Life & Casualty, author interview, March 1991.

31. Edward J. Kuriansky, deputy attorney general of New York State and special prosecutor for Medicaid fraud control, interview, February 1991.

32. *Time,* November 25, 1991.

33. The Health Insurance Association of America.

Chapter Four: The Politics of Reform

1. Barbara Ehrenreich and John Ehrenreich, editors, *The American Health Empire: Power, Profits and Politics* (New York: Random House, 1970).

2. Employee Benefit Research Institute.

3. The Jackson Hole Group, author interview, August 1993.

4. William M. Rodney, M.D., professor and chairman, Department of Family Medicine, University of Tennessee, Memphis, interviews, July and August 1993.

5. Richard Scott, chief executive officer, Columbia / HCA Healthcare, interview, November 1993.

Chapter Five: Jackson Who?

1. Paul M. Ellwood, M.D., interview, August 1993.

2. Paul M. Ellwood, M.D., interview, September 1993.

3. Robert Levine, "Rethinking Our Social Strategies," *The Public Interest,* Winter 1968, p. 88.

4. Richard D. Lyons, "Nixon's Health Care Plan Viewed as Replacing Chaotic Situation with Efficient System," *New York Times,* March 27, 1970.

5. Paul M. Ellwood, M.D., interview, June 1993.

6. Alain C. Enthoven, Marriner S. Eccles Professor of Public and Private Management, Stanford University, interview, December 1993.

7. Ibid.

8. Paul M. Ellwood, M.D., interview, May 1993.

9. John C. Lewin, M.D., director, Department of Health, State of Hawaii, interview, September 1993.

10. Edmund Faltermayer, "Where Doctors Scramble for Patients' Dollars," *Fortune,* November 6, 1978.

11. Paul M. Ellwood, M.D., interview, August 1993.

Chapter Six: The Clinton Plan

1. American Medical Association.

2. Congressman Jim Cooper, 4th District, Tennessee, interview, December 1993.

3. The Health Security Act, Title IV, Subtitle C.

4. Robert Pear, "Health Plan Leans on the Employers," *New York Times,* December 16, 1993.

5. The Health Security Act, Title VII, Subtitle A.

6. Congressman Jim Cooper, interview, December 1993.

Chapter Seven: Those Endless Costs

1. "Substance Abuse: The Nation's Number One Health Problem."

2. Ibid.

3. The Center on Addiction and Substance Abuse at Columbia University, July 1993.

4. Health Policy International, Princeton, New Jersey, 1993.

5. The Center on Addiction and Substance Abuse at Columbia University, July 1993.

6. The Children's Aid Society.

7. The Robert Wood Johnson Foundation, Princeton, New Jersey, 1993.

8. Natalie Davis Spingarn, *Hanging in There: Living Well on Borrowed Time* (New York: Stein and Day, 1982), p. 103.

9. Kirk Johnson, senior vice president and general counsel, American Medical Association, interview, September 1993.

Chapter Eight: Someone Else's Money

1. Paul Starr, *The Social Transformation of American Medicine* (New York: Basic Books, 1982), p. 295.

2. Ibid., p. 350.

3. Quoted in Paul M. Ellwood, M.D., "Program for Survival: A Proposed Course of Action for the Health Insurance Industry," paper presented October 5, 1967, before the Health Insurance Council, Denver, Colorado.

4. Ehrenreich and Ehrenreich, *The American Health Empire: Power, Profits and Politics*.

5. Employee Benefit Research Institute; U.S. Bureau of the Census.

6. K. Swartz and D. Lipson, "Strategies for Assisting the Medically Uninsured," the Urban Institute and the Intergovernmental Health Policy Project, Washington, D.C., 1989.

7. Milliman & Robertson, Inc.

8. Erik Eckholm, "Health Plan Is Toughest on Doctors Making Most," *New York Times*, November 7, 1993.

9. *New England Journal of Medicine*, September 30, 1993.

Chapter Nine: Why Doctors, Hospitals, and Drugs Cost So Much

1. American Medical Association.

2. The Medical Group Management Association, reported in Eckholm, "Health Plan Is Toughest on Doctors Making Most."

3. Dana Priest, "Hospital Bills Can Prove Hollow Basis for Health Care Comparisons," *Washington Post*, October 13, 1993.

4. American Hospital Association.

5. Pharmaceutical Manufacturers Association.

6. Boston Consulting Group, "The Changing Environment for U.S. Pharmaceuticals," April 1993.

7. *American Journal of Psychiatry*, November 1993.

8. R. N. Ross, et al., *Clinical Therapeutics*, 10(2): 188–203, 1988.

9. Charles A. Sanders, M.D., chairman and chief executive officer, Glaxo, interview, August 1993.

10. Boston Consulting Group, "The Changing Environment for U.S. Pharmaceuticals"; The Battelle Medical Technology and Policy Research Center.

11. William C. Steere, Jr., chairman and chief executive officer, Pfizer, Inc., interview, August 1993.

12. Philip Elmer-Dewitt, "The Genetic Revolution," *Time*, January 17, 1994.

13. Richard M. Weinshilboum, M.D., vice chair, board of trustees, Mayo Foundation, Mayo Clinic, interview, September 1993.

14. Pharmaceutical Manufacturers Association.

15. John Greenwald, "Ouch! Which Hurts More, the Shot or the Bill?" *Time*, March 8, 1993.

16. John C. Lewin, M.D., interviews, April 1992 and August 1993.

17. Milt Freudenheim, "A Drug Promotion Based on Price Breaks the Prescription Tradition," *New York Times,* November 9, 1993.

18. Brent James, M.D., executive director, Institute for Health Care Delivery Research, Intermountain Health Care, Salt Lake City, Utah, interview, November 12, 1993.

Chapter Ten: The Bean Counters: Insurance and Managed Care

1. Health Insurance Association of America.

2. American Hospital Association.

3. Bill Gradison, president, Health Insurance Association of America, Washington, D.C., interview, September 30, 1993.

4. Carl Schramm, "Economics," *Journal of the American Medical Association,* May 16, 1990.

5. Robert Pear, "Heads of HMOs Have Concerns on Health Plan," *New York Times,* October 18, 1993.

6. Stuart Gannes, "Strong Medicine For Health Bills," *Fortune,* April 13, 1987.

Chapter Eleven: Guaranteeing Quality

1. Daniel Callahan, president, the Hastings Center, interview, April 27, 1993.

2. Robert H. Brook, M.D., et al. "Predicting the Appropriate Use of Carotid Endarterectomy, Upper Gastrointestinal Endoscopy, and Coronary Angiography," *New England Journal of Medicine,* October 25, 1990, p. 1173.

3. Robert H. Brook, M.D., chairman, health sciences, Rand Corporation, interview, February 1992.

4. American Medical Association.

5. Ron Winslow, "Videos, Questionnaires Aim to Expand Role of Patients in Treatment Decisions," *Wall Street Journal,* February 25, 1992.

6. "Shared Decision-Making Programs," Foundation For Informed Medical Decision-Making, Dartmouth Medical School, 1993.

7. Paul M. Ellwood, M.D., interview, September 1993; Robert Brook, M.D., Santa Monica, California, interview, February 1994.

8. Greg Poulson, Susan Horn, Brent James, M.D., "Geographic Variation in Adjusted per Case Hospital Charges and Costs," Intermountain Health Care, Institute for Health Care Delivery Research, 1993.

9. Robert R. Waller, M.D., chief executive officer, Mayo Foundation, Mayo Clinic, interview, August 1993.

10. Robert R. Waller, M.D., interview, August 1993.

Chapter Twelve: How Other Countries Do It

1. Lee Smith, "A Cure for What Ails Medical Care," *Fortune*, July 1, 1991.

2. Health and Welfare Canada; The American Medical Association; U.S. Health Care Financing Administration.

3. Alain C. Enthoven, interview, December 1993.

4. Malcolm Gladwell, "Failing Health," *Saturday Night*, October 1993.

5. Joanna Miyake and Michael Walker, "Waiting Your Turn: Hospital Waiting Lists in Canada," Fraser Institute, Vancouver, British Columbia, May 1993.

6. Michael Walker, executive director, Fraser Institute, Vancouver, British Columbia.

7. Gladwell, "Failing Health."

8. Michael Walker, executive director, Fraser Institute, Vancouver, British Columbia, "Cold Reality: The Fraser Institute Survey of Physicians, 1991."

9. Eoin Kenny, "MPs, Senators and Top Bureaucrats Have Exclusive Medical Clinic," *Canadian Press*, September 17, 1993.

10. Consulate of Germany, New York, N.Y.

11. Ibid.

12. Manfred Stassen, "The German Statutory Health Insurance System," *Social Education*, September 1993.

13. Congressman Jim Cooper, interview, December 1993.

14. Kevin Grumbach, M.D., and John Fry, C.B.E., M.D., "Managing Primary Care in the United States and in the United Kingdom," *New England Journal of Medicine*, April 1, 1993.

15. Consulate of Australia, New York, N.Y.

16. William M. Rodney, M.D., interview, July 1993.

17. Jacques Krasny and Ian R. Ferrier, "The Canadian System in Perspective," Bogart Delafield Ferrier, Inc., July 1990.

18. Ibid.

19. Michael Walker, "The Other Side of Canada," letter to the editor, *Health Affairs*, Summer 1992.

20. Uwe Reinhardt, James Madison Professor of Economics, Princeton University, interview, July 1993.

Chapter Fourteen: All the King's Horses

1. Stephen Wiggins, chairman, Oxford Health Plans, interview, September 16, 1993.

2. M. Roy Schwarz, M.D., senior vice president for medical education and science, American Medical Association, Chicago, Illinois, interview, August 1993.

3. Richard M. Weinshilboum, M.D., vice chair, board of trustees,

Mayo Foundation, and director of education, Mayo Clinic, interview, September 1993.

4. Kirk Johnson, interview, September 1993.

5. Bill Gradison, interview, September 1993.

6. Robert R. Waller, M.D., interview, September 1993.

7. Alain C. Enthoven, interview, December 1993.

8. Ibid.

9. Howard Dean, M.D., governor of Vermont, interview, August 1993.

10. Brent James, interview, December 1993.

INDEX

273